How The Endocrine System Works

This new edition is also available as an e-book.
For more details, please see
www.wlley.com/buy/9781118931486
or scan this QR code:

How The Endocrine System Works

SECOND EDITION

J. Matthew Neal, MD, MBA, CPE, FACP, FACE, FACPE

Executive Medical Director, Academic Affairs
Indiana University Health Ball Memorial Hospital
Muncie, Indiana

Professor of Clinical Medicine
Indiana University School of Medicine
Indianapolis, Indiana

Series Editor

Lauren Sompayrac, PhD

WILEY Blackwell

Library of Congress Cataloging-in-Publication Data

Names: Neal, J. Matthew, author.
Title: How the endocrine system works / J. Matthew Neal.
Description: Second edition. | Chichester, West Sussex ; Hoboken, NJ : John
    Wiley & Sons, Inc., 2016. | Series: The how it works series | Includes
    bibliographical references and index.
Identifiers: LCCN 2015040692 (print) | LCCN 2015042778 (ebook) | ISBN
    9781118931486 (paperback) | ISBN 9781118931479 (pdf) | ISBN 9781118931462
    (epub)
Subjects: LCSH: Endocrine glands–Physiology. | Endocrine glands–Diseases. |
    Hormones–Physiological effect. | BISAC: MEDICAL / Endocrinology & Metabolism.
Classification: LCC QP187 .N35 2016 (print) | LCC QP187 (ebook) | DDC
    612.4–dc23
LC record available at http://lccn.loc.gov/2015040692

A catalogue record for this book is available from the British Library.

Wiley also publishes its books in a variety of electronic formats. Some content that appears in print
may not be available in electronic books.

Cover image: STEVE GSCHMEISSNER/Gettyimages

Set in 9.5/13 in Palatino Lt Std by SPi Global, Chennai, India

1   2016

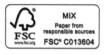

Contents

Acknowledgments, vii

How to Use this Book, ix

LECTURE 1   An Overview, 1

LECTURE 2   Pituitary and Hypothalamus, 13

LECTURE 3   The Thyroid, 25

LECTURE 4   Adrenal Gland, 39

LECTURE 5   Glucose Metabolism, 53

LECTURE 6   Calcium Metabolism, 77

LECTURE 7   Reproductive Endocrinology, 91

LECTURE 8   Lipid Disorders, 105

LECTURE 9   Disorders of Multiple Endocrine Glands and Paraneoplastic Syndromes, 115

APPENDIX   Clinical Trials, Evidence-Based Medicine, and Reading the Literature, 119

Glossary, 127

Index, 131

Acknowledgments

I am grateful to many individuals who were of assistance to me during the development of this book. I would like to thank the staff at Wiley-Blackwell, who asked me to revise this book and were very helpful during the development process. I am also very grateful to Dr Lauren Sompayrac, the editor of this series, who provided much feedback during the writing process. I would like to thank many of my residents and medical students who offered helpful advice and feedback. And, finally, I would like to thank my wife, Alexis, who was extremely helpful and patient during this revision.

How to Use this Book

I wrote this book as an overview of the endocrine system, and this is an update to my 2002 book of the same title. It is not intended for practising endocrinologists, but instead for those desiring a succinct introduction to this fascinating branch of medicine. It is also not meant to be a comprehensive text or examination study guide, as many such books are readily available. I wanted something that you could sit down with and readily assimilate in a few evenings, while providing sufficient background to apply the principles of endocrinology to your future clinical careers.

How The Endocrine System Works, Second Edition is written in a lecture format, as if I were talking to you personally. It is designed to be read from start to finish, and to be as entertaining as possible. (Some would dispute that endocrinology could ever be entertaining!) I have tried to interject some humor into the subject matter, and from time to time mention interesting historical events in endocrinology, such as the discovery of insulin and cortisone, as we can learn much from history. I have stressed the basics while avoiding excessive detail—as well as excessive simplicity.

A new addition to this update is a section on evidence-based medicine, epidemiology, and biostatistics, as any student of medicine needs to have an understanding of these principles. I have tried to present the information without boring you with too much detail.

Finally, review questions have been added to the end of each chapter.

This book may be used alone in an introductory course, or as a companion to a more detailed textbook. However you are using it, I hope that you enjoy it! Please feel free to provide any feedback to me regarding this text.

J. MATTHEW NEAL

LECTURE 1

An Overview

Endocrinology is the study of endocrine glands and their secretions. It can be a difficult topic to master because of all the mechanisms and feedback loops to understand. Yet, one way to understand the endocrine system is to break it down into smaller parts, and that is what I have attempted to accomplish in this book. It may help to visualize each endocrine system as part of a much larger group; envision a football team with all the players (quarterback, running backs, center, guards, receivers, punter, etc.). Each of these players must perform his job properly for the team to win. If even one player is out of sync, the play may be botched, even if the other players perform flawlessly. (In endocrinology, this happens frequently, as it does in other human disorders.) The quarterback is in charge of the team, calls the plays, and provides leadership. Hopefully your endocrine system has a good quarterback, but, as in football, some turn in lackluster performances, as do some supporting players.

Football teams often communicate plays with audible signals. Complex organisms also require detailed communication for proper function; they have developed hormones to send messages or commands from one part of the organism to another. Simple, one-celled organisms did not have a great need for detailed endocrine systems. But as organisms became more complex, large intercellular communication mechanisms became necessary for homeostasis.

The word "hormone" is derived from the Greek word meaning "arouse to activity." To many lay people, the word "hormone" conjures up images of estrogen or thyroid replacement therapy. In fact, there are many types of hormones, with new ones discovered every day; some have greater significance than others.

The endocrine system sends signals to the body by secreting hormones (e.g., insulin, growth hormone, thyroxine) directly into the circulation. In contrast, the exocrine glands secrete their substances into a duct system (e.g., sweat glands, exocrine pancreas).

The endocrine system is composed of many different glands throughout the body. The endocrine glands may be divided into two categories. The first, or "classical" glands' functions are primarily endocrine in nature. The second, or "nonclassical" glands' primary functions are something else, but they also secrete important substances.

The "classical" endocrine glands include the anterior pituitary, thyroid, parathyroids, adrenal cortex and medulla, gonads (testes and ovaries), and the endocrine pancreas. The primary function of these glands is to manufacture specific hormones. Some nonclassical endocrine organs and their hormones include the heart (atrial natriuretic peptide), kidney (calcitriol, renin), lymphocytes (cytokines, interleukins), GI tract (gastrin, secretin, vasoactive intestinal peptide), and many others. Many of the "classical" hormones are under the control of the hypothalamus and pituitary, which may be thought of as extensions of the nervous system. Indeed, the nervous and endocrine systems may function together quite closely (neuroendocrinology).

FUNCTION OF HORMONES

So why are hormones so important, anyway? The first thing that an organism must have in order to survive is energy. Food must be converted into energy, excess energy needs to be converted to storage, and stored energy must be mobilized when necessary to meet the organism's needs. In the chapter on glucose metabolism, we will learn the effects of insulin and glucagon on the body's metabolism and the many disorders where things go awry. Thyroid hormones are important in the regulation of the body's metabolism. Glycogen and lipids are necessary to provide long-term energy needs when food is not available.

The organism must maintain its internal environment. This is not as easy as it sounds. Many hormones play a role here. Hormones such as antidiuretic hormone, aldosterone, and atrial natriuretic peptide are important in water and sodium balance. Calcium is necessary for many bodily functions, and its metabolism is regulated by parathyroid hormone and vitamin D. Several hormones, including thyroid hormones, growth hormone, and sex steroids, control growth and development. These all need to work together as a team for the body to exist in an orderly environment.

And, of course, reproduction is essential for the continued survival of any organism. Specialized reproductive organs (gonads) produce sex steroids that are necessary for spermatogenesis and ovulation (as well as normal growth and development). Gonads are under the complex control of the hypothalamic–pituitary axis (HPA).

COMPOSITION OF HORMONES

Hormones are made from a variety of different molecules. The vast majority of hormones are of the protein or peptide variety. Proteins are chains of amino acids linked together. Some of these peptide hormones are only a few amino acids in length; most are much larger, with some being over 200 amino acids in length. Even the very small protein vasopressin (a nonapeptide) looks quite complex.

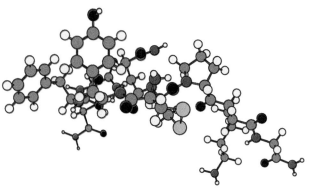

Arginine Vasopressin

Glycoproteins are sort of a hybrid hormone, consisting of a peptide hormone associated with a carbohydrate moiety. The four human glycoprotein hormones include LH (luteinizing hormone), FSH (follicle-stimulating hormone), TSH (thyroid-stimulating hormone or thyrotropin), and human chorionic gonadotropin (β-hCG). These hormones all share a common alpha subunit (α-SU); the β subunits differ from one to another.

Instead of being linked together to form proteins, one or two amino acids may be modified to form hormones. The amino acid tyrosine is modified to form the catecholamines (e.g., epinephrine and norepinephrine). While technically two amino acids joined together form a peptide, these amino acids are usually modified in some manner. The catecholamine hormones are very important in the nervous system. The thyroid or iodothyronine hormones (thyroxine, triiodothyronine) are made by joining two modified tyrosine molecules and adding several iodine atoms.

Tyrosine

Cholesterol, a molecule that we associate with atherosclerosis, is in fact essential to life. It is the precursor of steroid hormones—such as cortisol, aldosterone, estradiol, and testosterone—and sterol hormones, such as calcitriol.

OH
Cholesterol

Another common hormone precursor is the lowly fatty acid (the major storage component of fat), which serves as a precursor of hormones called eicosanoids. The most important eicosanoids, the prostaglandins, are derived from arachidonic acid. Other eicosanoids include thromboxanes, leukotrienes, and prostacyclins. They are important in smooth muscle contraction, hemostasis, inflammatory and immunologic responses, circulation, and respiratory and gastrointestinal systems.

Simple ions such as calcium also have hormone-like effects, and calcium metabolism will be discussed in Lecture 6.

HOW HORMONES WORK

Hormones must have a way to tell the other cells what to do. The end effect of a hormone is usually at the nucleus, resulting in the production of a protein that has some effect on the cell. Some hormones go directly to the nucleus and have an effect there. These types of hormones tend to be ones that can easily traverse the cell membrane; for this to happen, the hormone usually must be "nonpolar" (non-charged). These include the steroid and iodothyronine hormones.

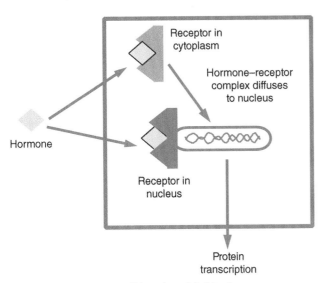

Hormones Interacting Directly with Nuclear or Cytoplasmic Receptors

The second class of hormones have no direct effect but instead bind to cell surface receptors, which initiates production of one or more second messengers that carry out the action. One messenger may trigger another messenger, which may trigger yet another, and so on. This concept of "multiple messengers" is called an amplification cascade and is the reason that some of these hormones are effective at extremely low concentrations (e.g., 10^{-12} mol/L). An analogy to the game of football would be a running back carrying the ball behind his blockers. Without the blockers, he is likely to be tackled quite quickly, ending the play abruptly; with multiple blockers, his power is "amplified" to the extent that many more yards can be gained than would have been possible alone. These hormones tend to be highly electrically charged, and include polypeptide, glycoprotein, and catecholamine hormones, and therefore cannot easily traverse the cell membrane.

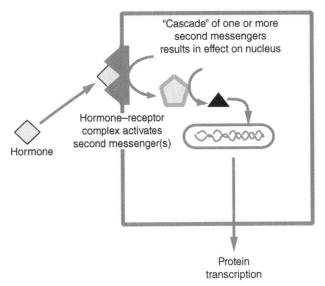

Hormones Interacting with Cell Surface Receptors

Another important difference between these hormones is how they travel in the blood. Those that act on the nucleus directly (e.g., steroids such as sex steroids (estradiol, testosterone, and glucocorticoids)) tend to travel bound to a carrier protein. (Interestingly, the mineralocorticoid steroids (e.g., aldosterone) do not have a binding protein.) These carrier proteins may be specific for those hormones (e.g., sex-hormone binding globulin, transcortin, thyroid-binding globulin), or may be common proteins (e.g., albumin). The hormones are often more slowly degraded if they are bound to carrier proteins, resulting in a longer half-life in serum.

The portion bound to the carrier protein is typically inactive. There is a small portion of the hormone that is not bound to the carrier protein, and this is called the active or free portion. This is clinically significant because some common conditions may result in an increase or decrease in the amount of carrier protein. This does not affect the free (active) portion, but does affect the total amount of hormone present (free + bound). Many laboratories measure the total, and not the free hormone level. Consequently, when there is a carrier protein abnormality, the total hormone may not accurately reflect the free level, which could lead to errors in diagnosis and management. Fortunately, many hormones can be measured in their free (unbound) state, which avoids this type of problem.

Peptide, glycoprotein, mineralocorticoid, and catecholamine hormones are not bound to carrier proteins and thus the type of problem mentioned above does not apply. Because they travel unbound in the plasma, they are usually degraded more quickly than the carrier-protein hormones. Some glycoproteins, because of their large carbohydrate component, are more slowly metabolized than pure peptide hormones.

HORMONAL REGULATION

Although endocrinology is very complex, the good thing is that much of it can be figured out if you understand the mechanisms. Most hormones have another hormone that regulates its secretion; a hormone that stimulates another hormone's secretion is called a trophic or stimulatory hormone. Those that cause less of the hormone to be secreted are called inhibitory hormones. The hormone thus secreted by the gland of interest causes a desired effect at the target gland's nucleus (e.g., production of a protein). Once this substance reaches a desired level, it tells the trophic hormone cells to slow down and stop stimulating the endocrine organ. This causes reduction in the hormone levels by a process called feedback inhibition. This keeps the whole system in check by preventing too much hormone from being synthesized. In effect, the end product of the endocrine organ becomes a type of indirect inhibitory hormone (by decreasing production of the trophic hormone).

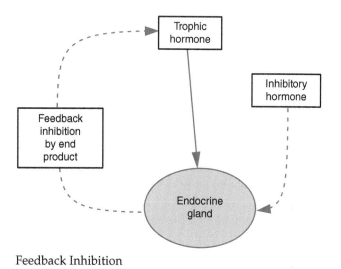

Feedback Inhibition

You may compare the concept of feedback inhibition to filling up your car with gas. You go to the gas station when your gauge says that the tank is empty. Problems may arise when the gauge malfunctions (e.g., you have a full tank when it reads empty, or vice versa, resulting in inadvertently running out of fuel). When you fill up the tank, the pump should stop delivering gas when the tank is full. If it stops too soon, the tank will not be full; if it does not stop after the tank is full, gas spills out all over the place. The purpose of feedback inhibition is to keep the "gas tank" at the correct level.

When something disrupts the normal feedback mechanisms, the endocrine system goes awry and hormonal abnormalities result. Most endocrine disorders can be understood by thinking of ways that the feedback mechanisms become disordered, resulting in disruption of the endocrine system:

1. Target organ is damaged or absent and produces insufficient hormone (hypofunction), despite normal stimulatory pathways: it cannot respond to trophic hormone stimulation (primary deficiency, such as hypothyroidism due to Hashimoto's thyroiditis or thyroidectomy; i.e., the organ is damaged or absent).
2. Target organ produces too much hormone (hyperfunction—the gas pump does not stop despite the tank being full): autonomous secretion of hormone occurs despite suppressed trophic hormone (e.g., Cushing's syndrome [cortisol hypersecretion] due to autonomously functioning adrenal tumor; hyperthyroidism due to toxic nodular goiter).
3. Receptor defect/hormone resistance: desired effect not produced despite the presence of large amounts of hormone (e.g., type 2 diabetes mellitus, androgen insensitivity syndrome (testicular feminization)).
4. Excess trophic hormone that secondarily produces excess target organ hormone (e.g., Cushing's syndrome due to excess corticotropin [ACTH] production).
5. Deficiency of trophic hormone: inadequate target organ hormone produced despite structurally intact primary organ (secondary deficiency, e.g., hypopituitarism).
6. Administration of excess exogenous hormone (e.g., Cushing's syndrome due to excess corticosteroid administration).

INTERACTIONS BETWEEN THE ENDOCRINE AND IMMUNE SYSTEMS

It was recognized long ago that alterations in the immune system occur after a significant change in the endocrine milieu (e.g., gonadectomy, pregnancy). This led to the proposition that there are important interactions between the immune and endocrine systems. Cytokines are extremely potent molecules secreted by immune cells that have significant regulatory effects on the endocrine system; in a way, they act as hormones themselves. Hundreds of different cytokines have been isolated, and include the interleukins, tumor necrosis factors, interferons, transforming growth factors, and colony-stimulating factors. Such immune factors may either inhibit or potentiate endocrine secretion. For example, it was observed long ago that severe burn victims increased their corticosteroid and catecholamine production dramatically; much of this increase can be explained by the effects of various inflammatory factors on the adrenal cortex and medulla. A very common condition called the euthyroid sick syndrome appears to be at least partially mediated by inflammatory products such as cytokines. A full discussion of this topic is complex and beyond the scope of this text.

HORMONE MEASUREMENTS

Although we can measure most known hormones in the blood, the circumstances under which we measure them are very important. Random hormone levels are often of little use because many hormones are secreted in periodic or cyclical manner, with levels varying throughout the day. For example, cortisol levels are typically highest in the morning, but lower in the evening. These levels are often the opposite in a person who works the "night shift." Totally blind individuals sometimes lose this cyclical variation, so it appears that the presence of daylight may have some influence on this phenomenon.

To adequately study secretion of some hormones, we must perform a "perturbation" study in which a substance is given to produce a desired result (i.e., stimulation or inhibition of the hormone's secretion). If one is concerned about hormone deficiency, a stimulatory test is done by administering a secretagogue (substance that provokes a hormonal response). The hormone of interest is usually measured before, and at one or more intervals after, administration of the secretagogue.

If hormonal excess is instead suspected, then a suppression or inhibitory test is performed: a substance known to suppress hormone levels is administered. For example, random growth hormone (GH) levels are often not useful in evaluating GH excess (gigantism or acromegaly) because of the episodic secretion of pituitary hormones. Since hyperglycemia is a known inhibitor of GH secretion, a glucose suppression test is possible, in which GH levels are measured before and after a large oral glucose load. In normal health, GH is suppressed; in acromegaly, secretion is autonomous and it is not suppressed.

An alternative to a provocative test may be urine collection over a long period of time (e.g., 24 h), which eliminates some of the problems associated with random hormone measurements. For example, pheochromocytomas often secrete catecholamines intermittently, making random measurements suboptimal during a quiescent period. A 24-h urine collection for catecholamines and metabolites will usually be elevated in these persons (although plasma measurements may be useful during active episodes).

One must often use caution in the interpretation of laboratory test "normal values." Most human measurements (height, weight, intelligence, etc.) and measurements of hormone function follow the normal distribution or "bell curve":

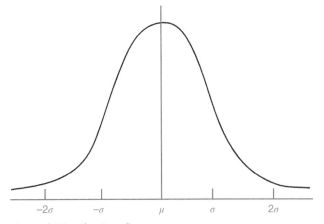

Normal Distribution Curve

The normal distribution curve is symmetrical about the mean (μ) or 50th percentile. One and two standard deviations (σ) above the mean correspond approximately to the 84th and 97.5th percentiles, respectively; one and two standard deviations below the mean correspond to the 16th and 2.5th percentiles, respectively. A laboratory often defines "normal ranges" as a 95% confidence interval (two standard deviations above and below the mean); this means that by definition, 5% of "normal" persons fall outside the "normal range," and that minimally abnormal values may simply represent a normal variant.

Normal ranges may vary according to variations in population (age, gender, ethnicity, etc.). For example, "normal" TSH levels in pregnancy are significantly lower than in nonpregnant females, due to the high concentration of the glycoprotein hormone β-hCG, which has TSH-like activity at the very high concentrations found in pregnancy (so less native TSH is needed); in addition, "normal" TSH values are higher in elderly patients. Hemoglobin A_{1c} levels (an index of long-term glycemic control in diabetes) appear to be slightly higher in African Americans and Hispanic Americans (given equivalent glucose levels), due to genetic factors not related to glucose control.

In addition, "normal ranges" for some hormones may be quite wide, for example, the normal range for serum total thyroxine is approximately 5.0–12.0 µg/dL. So, it is possible for a person to have hypothyroidism with a "normal" T4 of 5.2 µg/dL; "normal" for him or her might really be 9 µg/dL. It is often useful, therefore, to measure both the hormone of interest and the trophic hormone (called a "hormone pair"). Indeed, many patients with low normal T4 levels have elevated TSH levels, indicating mild primary ("subclinical") hypothyroidism. Measuring the pair often yields more information than either hormone measurement provides alone.

NOMENCLATURE OF ENDOCRINE DISORDERS

A normal endocrine state is denoted by the Greek prefix "eu" (e.g., euglycemia, euthyroid, eucalcemic). Hypofunctional states contain the prefix "hypo" (e.g., hypoparathyroidism, hypopituitarism); the prefix "hyper" means too much, obviously. Examples of hyperfunctional states include hyperthyroidism, hyperparathyroidism, and hyperinsulinism. These disorders

may be classified more specifically. For example, there are many causes of hyperthyroidism: Graves' disease, toxic nodular goiter, and subacute thyroiditis. Patients with elevated glucose levels are usually said to have diabetes mellitus rather than hyperglycemia.

HYPOFUNCTION

Hormone deficiency syndromes

Endocrine deficiency occurs if the primary (target) organ functions inadequately or is absent; this is a primary deficiency disorder. Examples include hypothyroidism due to Hashimoto's thyroiditis or thyroidectomy, Addison's disease (primary adrenal insufficiency), and type 1 diabetes mellitus. In primary disorders, the organ's trophic hormone level is elevated; for example, those with primary hypothyroidism have an elevated serum TSH level. The trophic hormone in this case is "beating a dead horse"—the gland does not work properly despite massive attempts to stimulate it.

Secondary deficiency disorders occur when the trophic hormone for the target organ is deficient. This occurs in hypopituitarism, in which the target organs (thyroid, adrenal, gonads) are structurally intact, but are not stimulated properly. Tertiary disorders are similar to secondary syndromes except that the deficiency is one step higher; that is, the trophic hormone for the trophic gland is deficient. An example is hypothalamic dysfunction, in which the hypothalamic hormones are made in insufficient amounts to stimulate the pituitary, and in turn, the target organs.

Antibody-mediated (autoimmune) endocrine organ destruction is the most common cause of hormone deficiency. Our bodies normally produce antibodies to defend against invaders such as viruses and bacteria. Occasionally, however, the body may produce antibodies that attack its own organs, causing destruction. The tendency for autoimmune diseases is genetically mediated, but environmental factors (i.e., exposure to an environmental "trigger"—perhaps an antigen that triggers an antibody response) seem to be a requirement as well.

Inflammatory or infiltrative disease may also result in organ destruction and hormone deficiency. Patients with inflammation of the pancreas (pancreatitis) may develop diabetes due to insufficient insulin secretion. Hemochromatosis is a relatively common genetic disorder of iron overload in which excessive iron deposits cause organ dysfunction. This disorder may cause diabetes and adrenal insufficiency.

Large tumors in or about the target organ may destroy enough cells to cause hormone deficiency. A common example is pituitary hormone deficiency (hypopituitarism), which is often caused by the destructive effects of very large pituitary or suprasellar tumors. Destructive tumors more commonly cause secondary rather than primary endocrine deficiencies.

Hormone resistance

It is also possible for a hormone to be made in sufficient quantity, but to have inadequate effect because of resistance to the hormone. Here, the patient's hormone receptors are either absent or insufficiently sensitive to the hormone for the desired metabolic effect to occur. This appears to the clinician as a true endocrine deficiency disorder, even though normal or even increased amounts of the hormone are made. The most common example is type 2 diabetes mellitus, in which patients are (in initial stages) insulin resistant. These patients develop elevated blood glucose levels (hyperglycemia), despite normal or even high levels of serum insulin. Very large amounts of exogenous insulin may be required to overcome the insulin resistance.

TREATMENT OF HORMONE DEFICIENCY

Ideally, we treat deficiency syndromes by replacing the native hormone, producing normal physiologic levels. This is pretty easy for orally absorbed molecules that have a relatively long half-life (e.g., thyroxine, hydrocortisone, estradiol). Some hormones, however, are not well absorbed orally. These include most peptide hormones, which are destroyed by acids and digestive enzymes in the gastrointestinal tract. Many of these are given by injection; examples include insulin and growth hormone. Some peptides are synthetically modified to have a longer duration in the blood; these include desmopressin (a derivative of antidiuretic hormone or vasopressin which can be given orally) and octreotide (an analog of somatostatin given subcutaneously).

Other hormones such as testosterone are well absorbed orally, but are metabolized in the liver to inactive products (the "first-pass" phenomenon) before they get to the circulation, rendering them inert. These hormones must be given by injection, intranasally, or via transdermal (gel or patch) preparation.

And, even if we have the hormone to provide, it may not be possible to replace it in a precise physiological manner. The best example of this is type 1 diabetes mellitus, in which the patient is dependent on insulin injections to sustain life. Despite many technological advances, it is currently impossible to mimic insulin secretion perfectly. At best, the patient must learn to live with compromises, such as occasional hyperglycemia and hypoglycemia, which may interfere with daily living.

ENDOCRINE EXCESS SYNDROMES

As with deficiency syndromes, excess may occur in primary or secondary forms. A primary disorder occurs when the organ itself produces the excess hormone without stimulation by a trophic gland. An example is primary hyperaldosteronism caused by an autonomous adrenal tumor. A common example of a secondary excess syndrome is Cushing's disease, which is caused by increased production of adrenocorticotropic hormone (ACTH) by a pituitary tumor. In this case, there is nothing wrong with the target organ (the adrenal gland)—it is responding as it should to excess trophic hormone. The "wide receiver" (adrenal cortex) is simply obeying the quarterback (pituitary), who has "called the wrong play."

Unlike hormone deficiency (usually caused by autoimmune diseases), hormone excess syndromes are typically caused by tumors (benign or malignant). These tumors typically arise in the organ that normally produces the hormone. Hyperfunctioning tumors may also arise in an organ other than the one normally producing the hormone; these conditions are called paraneoplastic or ectopic ("out of place") syndromes. We will discuss these syndromes in the final lecture.

Autoimmune syndromes only rarely cause endocrine excess as part of rather esoteric syndromes. An exception is the common condition Graves' disease, where thyroid receptor autoantibodies mimic the trophic hormone (TSH) and result in hyperthyroidism.

Another reason for hormone excess is exogenous administration of the hormone, either intentionally (iatrogenic) or by the patient without the physician's knowledge (factitious). For example, glucocorticoids are commonly used to treat transplant patients to prevent rejection. Chronic administration in past high-steroid regimens resulted in iatrogenic Cushing's syndrome. (Fortunately, current immunosuppressive regimens today use very low steroid doses and depend on the immune-modifying actions of newer drugs targeting specific aspects of the immune process, mostly eliminating these problems.) Glucocorticoids are still used in high doses at times to treat other chronic diseases (e.g., rheumatologic and pulmonary disease).

An example of factitious hormone use is the person who wishes to lose weight by taking exogenous thyroid hormone (not prescribed by any physician), or those without diabetes who self-induce hypoglycemia with insulin or sulfonylureas. These cases are often health care workers with psychiatric problems and access to medication.

IMAGING TESTS IN ENDOCRINOLOGY

Plain X-rays (roentgenograms) are inexpensive and simple to perform, but have limited use in endocrinology. At the energy levels used for imaging, X-rays are absorbed to a great extent by molecules containing elements with high atomic numbers (Z, or number of protons in the nucleus). Such molecules appear opaque (white) on X-ray. Iodine ($Z = 53$) and barium ($Z = 56$) are relatively heavy elements, which is why they are commonly used as radiocontrast agents. (This use of stable iodine has nothing to do with the uses of its radioactive counterparts.) Molecules containing calcium ($Z = 20$) also show up well on X-ray (think of bones, which are quite dense). Some endocrine disorders are associated with ectopic calcification and may be detected on plain X-ray. Conversely, organic molecules predominantly contain carbon, oxygen, nitrogen, sulfur, phosphorus, and hydrogen (low atomic number elements) and are thus not visualized well on conventional X-ray films.

Nuclear medicine imaging studies use radioactive substances that are administered to patients. They may be given orally (e.g., radioiodine), intravenously (technetium sulfur colloid), or inhaled (xenon). The element used is typically a radioactive counterpart (isotope) of a nonradioactive element (or one with similar chemical properties). For example, ^{123}I and ^{131}I are isotopes of the nonradioactive (stable) [127]I. (The superscript immediately preceding the chemical symbol indicates the mass number (A), which is the number of protons (Z) plus the number of neutrons.) Other elements do not occur in the natural compound but are similar in structure and chemical properties to the natural element. Technetium (^{99m}Tc) is a synthetic transition metal with radioactive properties making it very suitable for imaging. It is the lowest atomic number element ($Z = 43$) without any stable isotopes, and lies in the periodic table between molybdenum and ruthenium. Its low toxicity, ease of incorporation into numerous compounds, and low cost make it an all-purpose versatile radionuclide. In nuclear studies, the radioactive element is either administered in its native form or attached to a molecule that mimics the native substance.

Radionuclides may emit radiation in several ways. They may emit non-particulate energy such as photons (gamma rays), which are essentially high-energy light beams. Gamma radiation occurs after a nuclear event (e.g., β decay) that leaves the nucleus in an excited state. When the nucleus returns to its unexcited (ground) state, gamma rays are emitted from the nucleus. X-rays are exactly the same type of energy as gamma rays except that their origin is the outer electron shells rather than the nucleus when an electron passes from a higher to a lower energy state. Iodine-123 (^{123}I) and technetium are examples of pure gamma emitters.

Some radionuclides emit particulate radiation in addition to gamma rays. The nuclides of clinical interest emit beta (β) particles, which are electrons ejected from the nucleus, resulting in conversion of a neutron to a proton. β-Particles may cause significant tissue destruction, and therefore these elements are less suitable for imaging. They are used when actual destruction of tissue is desired. [131]I is a powerful β emitter used to destroy thyroid tissue in those with hyperthyroidism and thyroid cancer. Heavy nuclides that emit α particles (e.g., thorium, uranium, and radium) have no real clinical use in nuclear medicine. Some α-emitters have therapeutic use in targeted radioimmunotherapy.

Radionuclides disintegrate because of the very properties that make them radioactive; the half-life is the amount of time for half of the nuclide to disintegrate. Decay is exponential and the amount present at any time can be calculated if the half-life and original amount of the radionuclide are known:

$$A = A_0 e^{\frac{-0.693t}{t_{1/2}}}$$

where A = activity of the nuclide at the current time; A_0 = original activity of nuclide; t = time elapsed; $t_{1/2}$ = half-life of nuclide; and e = base of the natural logarithm (2.71828 …).

The physical amount of a radionuclide is denoted by its activity and is proportional to the number of disintegrations per second. The traditional unit of radionuclide activity is the curie (named after Marie

Curie, a prominent nuclear physicist and discoverer of polonium and radium). The amounts used in nuclear medicine are in the range of 1/1,000th curie (millicurie, mCi) or 1/1,000,000th curie (microcurie, µCi). Another unit of activity (used more commonly outside the United States) is the becquerel (Bq); 1 mCi = 37 MBq (megabecquerels). While activity (mCi or MBq) refers to an actual physical amount of radionuclide, the delivered dose of radiation depends on many factors, such as type of energy emitted and energy of the gamma rays, and is beyond the scope of this text. For example, 30 mCi of ^{131}I delivers approximately 100 times as much radiation as 30 mCi of ^{123}I because of the increased energy and particulate emissions of the former.

A radiation counter can detect the amount of gamma radiation emitted. It merely measures the amount of radiation coming from the patient and provides no spatial information. A radionuclide uptake may be calculated using these measurements to provide the fractional amount of nuclide accumulated at a given time. A more complex device, a gamma camera, can produce a two-dimensional image or scan of the organ radiating the energy. Gamma cameras are used to produce thyroid scan images, for example. Although nuclear medicine provides useful functional information, the scan resolution is typically far less than other imaging modalities.

Ultrasound utilizes high-frequency sound waves and takes advantage of their attenuation by various materials. Sound waves are generated by a transducer and placed in contact with the body. The sound is either reflected back to the transducer or absorbed. The distance between the transducer and the reflected echo is calculated by measuring the time between the transmitted wave and the echo. The material that absorbs sound (e.g., air) transmits little or no sound back to the transducer. Very sophisticated images can be obtained by using multiple transducers; high-speed computers collect and interpret the data in a two-dimensional form that can be displayed on a screen.

Unlike nuclear medicine, ultrasound does not expose the patient to ionizing radiation. It is also a "real-time" modality that can be used to guide procedures (e.g., fine-needle aspiration biopsy or insertion of a catheter into a difficult area). The resolution of ultrasound, however, is less than that of magnetic resonance imaging (MRI) or computed tomography (CT). Nor is ultrasound very useful for air-filled cavities (e.g., lung).

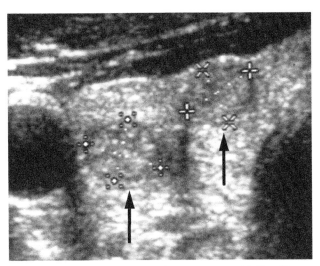

Ultrasound of Thyroid Nodule in Patient with Papillary Thyroid Carcinoma

Computed tomography (CT) uses conventional X-ray beams to produce high-resolution "cross-sections" of a body part. The patient is placed between the X-ray tube and a series of X-ray detectors, which move in a circular manner around the patient. After the detectors have completed a full circle around the patient, the data is analyzed by a computer, which reconstructs an image, a virtual "cross-section" of the area of interest. A recent development is the high-resolution (helical or spiral) CT, in which the X-ray tube and detectors move in a helical manner from one end of the area to the other, resulting in many more data points than conventional CT. Single-photon emission computed tomography (SPECT) is a hybrid of CT and nuclear medicine that uses an administered nuclear source rather than an X-ray beam for the radiation source.

Because of its speed, CT is useful for imaging large body cavities (e.g., chest, abdomen, or pelvis) that contain visceral organs. Iodine-containing contrast agents are often administered to help identify key structures. These are contraindicated in those with renal insufficiency. Many patients are allergic and require pretreatment with corticosteroids and antihistamines. These agents also interfere with radioiodine imaging of the thyroid for at least 4 weeks.

MRI takes advantage of the effect of hydrogen nuclei when exposed to a strong magnetic field. At rest, the nuclei are oriented at random. When exposed to a magnetic field, the nuclei "polarize" and oscillate at a certain frequency that is unique to each atom. Since the body is about 80% water (H_2O), there is a lot of hydrogen to polarize. Sophisticated computer reconstruction of these faint MR signals results in detailed cross-sectional images of the body. A greater variety of imaging angles is available with MRI than CT. Another advantage is the lack of ionizing radiation. A disadvantage is the relatively long scan times compared to CT. The patient must often be enclosed, which may be difficult for those with claustrophobia. "Open" MRI units now exist in which the patient is only partially enclosed. These devices use weaker magnets, however, and may be less suitable for precise imaging of very small structures such as the pituitary. MRI strength is expressed in tesla (T) units. A unit with strength of 0.5 T is relatively weak, while the strongest units have magnetic fields up to 6 T.

Positron emission tomography (PET) uses short-lived radionuclides such as fluorine-18, which can be incorporated into compounds used by the body, such as glucose; PET can therefore measure metabolic activity in tissues in addition to providing anatomic information. A positron is an electron with a positive charge. When a positron and electron strike each other, they are converted to energy by an "annihilation reaction," which can be detected by sensors. PET has been used primarily to measure cerebral and myocardial blood flow, but has shown promise in certain endocrine applications (e.g., detection of thyroid cancer metastases). A disadvantage of PET is the extremely short half-lives of the radionuclides, mandating that they be made at the facility in a cyclotron. Another is the expense (due to the high cost of the radionuclides and equipment, it is one of the most expensive diagnostic tests available).

GENETIC TESTING IN ENDOCRINOLOGY

When insulin was discovered in the 1920s (a remarkable achievement), no one understood much about human genetics, other than the obvious (tall parents tend to have tall children, baldness runs in the family, etc.). It would be another 30 years before DNA was discovered (early 1950s), and decades before that was completely understood. To think that today we would be able to determine molecular genetic markers of disease would seem incomprehensible at that time. Yet, the number of available biomarkers increases at a rapid pace as technology develops at an exponential rate.

The discovery of new genetic markers makes it easier to diagnose diseases earlier and treat before symptoms develop. For example, family members of patients with multiple endocrine neoplasia (MEN) II once had to undergo cumbersome testing procedures for the disorders

Examples of Genetic Markers in Endocrinology

KAL-1, FGFR1	Kallmann syndrome
PHEX (phosphate-regulating endopeptidase homolog)	X-linked hypophosphatemic rickets
Glucokinase (GCK), hepatocyte nuclear factor 1α, KCNJ11	Maturity-onset diabetes of the young (MODY)
BRAF, PPARγ	Epithelial thyroid carcinoma
PROP1, POU1F1	Hypopituitarism
RET, VHL, SDHB	Familial pheochromocytoma/paraganglioma syndromes, multiple endocrine neoplasia II
MENIN	Multiple endocrine neoplasia I
SHOX (short stature homeobox)	Turner syndrome, other short stature syndromes

encountered in this syndrome (e.g., medullary thyroid carcinoma, pheochromocytoma). The importance of detection in potentially affected patients is immense in some circumstances (e.g., pheochromocytoma can be lethal if untreated). Instead of undergoing complex testing, measurement of the RET (rearranged during transfection) proto-oncogene can identify patients at risk, who can then undergo prophylactic surgery (e.g., thyroidectomy) if positive.

Most common endocrine diseases are still diagnosed by clinical rather than molecular genetic criteria. While some rare forms of diabetes are linked to specific genetic mutations, the most common form of type 2 diabetes is a heterogeneous disorder without identified genetic markers. The common autoimmune endocrine disorders (type 1 diabetes, Hashimoto's thyroiditis, etc.) are linked to specific HLA haplotypes, although the penetrance is variable; we know that, for a person to develop an autoimmune endocrine disease, some environmental "trigger" must be present, as genetics are not enough. For example, in monozygotic (identical) twins, the concordance rate of type 1 diabetes is only about 50%, meaning that there is an additional, nongenetic factor that must be present for the other twin to develop the disorder.

This is all good—but remember that genetic testing is quite expensive (>$1,000 per gene), although this cost may decrease in the future as technology improves. Therefore, it is practical today only to test patients in whom identification of a specific genetic defect would alter treatment or have impact on family members.

EPILOGUE

This lecture has laid the framework for discussion of the endocrine system. Hopefully, you now have a basic idea of how the different systems fit together. In the next several lectures, we will examine each of the "players" in detail, discussing previous lectures as needed. Finally, we will discuss disorders of multiple endocrine glands in the last lecture.

REVIEW QUESTIONS

1. A 27-year-old woman is in an automobile accident and suffers the complete transection of the pituitary stalk in a traumatic brain injury. She would have deficiency of all the following hormones except one:
   a. Estradiol
   b. Thyroxine
   c. Cortisol
   d. Aldosterone
   e. Growth hormone
   (d) Aldosterone secretion is regulated by the renin–angiotensin system, and not by the pituitary. All the others are dependent on normal pituitary function for proper secretion.

2. In which one of the following disorders is the deficient hormone itself not used in treatment?
   a. Hypoparathyroidism
   b. Type 1 diabetes mellitus
   c. Primary adrenal insufficiency
   d. Primary hypogonadism
   e. Primary hypothyroidism
   (a) While synthetic PTH is available as a treatment for osteoporosis, it is not used for the treatment of hypoparathyroidism. The others are treated with insulin, glucocorticoids/mineralocorticoids, sex steroids, and thyroxine, respectively.

3. In which one of the following disorders is the target organ hormone of interest *elevated* rather than *decreased*?
   a. Hypoparathyroidism
   b. Primary hypothyroidism due to Hashimoto's thyroiditis
   c. Primary hypothyroidism due to orchidectomy
   d. Type 1 diabetes mellitus
   e. Type 2 diabetes mellitus
   (e) Type 2 diabetes (at least in its early stages) is a disorder of hormone resistance (to insulin, in this case), and not of deficiency. Despite elevated levels of insulin, receptor defects do not allow proper function. The others are clear cases of hormone deficiency.

4. Suppressive or inhibitory tests are usually done to evaluate endocrine excess. Which one of the following is a stimulatory or provocative test used primarily to evaluate endocrine deficiency?
   a. Dexamethasone test
   b. Cosyntropin (synthetic ACTH) test
   c. Saline infusion test
   d. Glucose tolerance test
   (b) Cosyntropin (1–24 ACTH) stimulates the adrenal cortex to produce cortisol, and is useful in the evaluation of adrenal insufficiency. Dexamethasone (a) is used in suppressive tests for evaluation of Cushing's syndrome; saline infusion suppresses aldosterone levels and is used in the evaluation of hyperaldosteronism; glucose (d) suppresses growth hormone levels and is employed in the evaluation of growth hormone excess (gigantism and acromegaly).

5. Which one of the following patients does not have a primary endocrine deficiency disorder?
   a. A 52-year-old woman going through menopause
   b. A 34-year-old man who has a thyroidectomy for thyroid cancer
   c. A 16-year-old girl with new onset diabetes mellitus requiring insulin
   d. A 14-year-old boy with hypopituitarism due to an intracranial tumor
   e. A 47-year-old male with HIV and adrenal insufficiency due to adrenal fungal infection
   (d) This patient has multiple secondary endocrine deficiencies (hypothyroidism, adrenal insufficiency, hypogonadism, etc.) due to lack of pituitary trophic hormones. The others are examples of primary deficiency disorders.

LECTURE 2

Pituitary and Hypothalamus

REVIEW

Let us quickly review the first lecture. We learned that complex multicellular organisms require a way to regulate bodily functions by communicating between cells. This is accomplished by means of the endocrine system, in which a substance (hormone) secreted by one type of cell may have an effect on a cell far away, in a different part of the body. Hormones are necessary for cellular communication and regulation in highly evolved organisms. If hormone levels get "out of whack," the body does not function at optimal efficiency, and can even perish in some cases. Most hormones are proteins made of tens to hundreds of amino acids. Others are modified amino acids (catecholamines, iodothyronines) or derivatives of cholesterol (steroids). Glycoproteins are a special type of protein hormone to which large sugar molecules are attached.

Each hormone has a desired effect on a target cell. The effect may be stimulatory (to cause the cell to produce a substance—usually a protein), or inhibitory (to inhibit production of the substance). Production of this substance in the target cell takes place in the nucleus. Some hormones go to the nucleus directly and have their effect there; other hormones attach to the cell membrane and trigger production of one or more second messengers that travel to the nucleus and produce the desired effect. A multiple-messenger "cascade" allows extremely low concentrations of these hormones to have a significant effect. Some hormones travel in serum bound to carrier proteins—others travel in the free state.

Understanding hormonal regulation is essential for understanding endocrinology. Most hormones have another hormone that regulates their secretion, and those that stimulate a hormone's secretion are called trophic hormones. Those that inhibit are called inhibitory

hormones. A trophic hormone has a target gland and once the target gland hormone reaches a normal level, feedback inhibition on the trophic gland keeps levels from becoming too high. In a way, the target hormone becomes a sort of indirect inhibitory hormone. All endocrine disorders result from disruption of the normal feedback mechanisms.

Endocrine hypofunction is common and is typically caused by an abnormal or absent gland (a primary deficiency). Autoimmune gland destruction is the most common cause of primary endocrine hypofunction. Less common are the secondary and tertiary causes of hypofunction, in which deficient trophic hormones result in inadequate target gland function. A target organ's resistance to the trophic hormone may also cause hypofunction. In most cases of organ hypofunction, we try and replace the native hormone. However, this is not possible or practical in some instances, as it may be simpler to administer the target organ hormone. And, even if we have the hormone, it may be difficult to replace it in the exact physiologic manner (e.g., diabetes).

In contrast to organ hypofunction, most cases of endocrine hyperfunction are caused by tumors, while autoimmune causes of hyperfunction are rare. Another cause of endocrine excess is the exogenous administration of a hormone in supraphysiologic doses (e.g., thyroid hormone or glucocorticoids).

Some hormones may be measured in their basal state. Many, however, are secreted periodically, and random measurement may not be useful. When endocrine hypofunction is suspected, we often perform a stimulatory test by giving the trophic hormone to the patient; the response to the stimulus is then measured. If we suspect endocrine excess, an inhibitory test is performed by administering a feedback inhibitor of the hormone to see if the target hormone decreases appropriately.

Many imaging tests are useful in endocrinology. Plain X-rays are inexpensive but have limited value in endocrinology other than surveying the skeleton. Nuclear medicine involves the administration of radioactive substances that are assimilated into compounds inside the body. The radiation source therefore is the patient, and radiation counts and/or images may be obtained to assess function. Most nuclear medicine studies in endocrinology use radioactive iodine. One type of radioiodine (iodine-123) is very useful for imaging, while another type (iodine-131) is more useful for destroying thyroid tissue. Technetium, a synthetic radioactive element, is also important in nuclear medicine imaging due to its low toxicity and ease of incorporation into many compounds.

Computed tomography (CT) utilizes conventional X-rays to produce cross-sections of an organ. Magnetic resonance imaging (MRI) uses powerful magnetic fields to produce cross-sectional images as well. MRI provides better resolution of some endocrine structures (e.g., pituitary) than does CT. Ultrasound utilizes the attenuation of high-frequency sound waves by an organ to provide a real-time image. Advantages of MRI and ultrasound include the absence of ionizing radiation.

PITUITARY AND HYPOTHALAMUS

In this chapter we will discuss the "master glands": the pituitary and the hypothalamus. In our football team analogy, they are sort of like the "quarterback" that directs the rest of the glands. (Not every gland is controlled by the pituitary and hypothalamus; think of these other glands as "special teams" glands.) In fact, the pituitary and hypothalamus tend to function together as 1 unit, which we will call the hypothalamic–pituitary axis (HPA), and which serves to integrate the central nervous system and the endocrine system. Most of the "classical" endocrine glands are under control of the HPA.

The pituitary is a small gland that lies in a part of the skull called the sella turcica, at the base of the skull. It is divided into the anterior lobe (adenohypophysis) and the posterior lobe (neurohypophysis). The anterior lobe cells manufacture what we normally think of as the pituitary hormones. Their secretion is influenced by hypothalamic hormones that travel to the anterior lobe via a humoral system called the hypophyseal portal system.

The anterior pituitary makes hormones that control specific glands, which include:

ACTH (adrenocorticotrophic hormone or corticotropin)—adrenal cortex
GH (growth hormone or somatotropin)—bone and muscle
PRL (prolactin)—milk-producing glands of breast

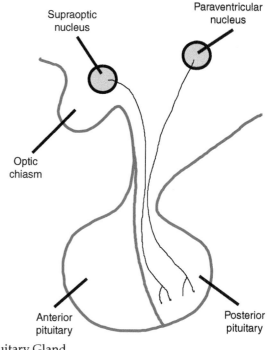

Pituitary Gland

TSH (thyroid-stimulating hormone or thyrotropin)—thyroid
LH (luteinizing hormone) and FSH (follicle-stimulating hormone)—ovaries and testes.

The hypothalamus is a group of neurons in the midbrain that secretes a variety of substances. The hypothalamic hormones can be divided into two types. The first are those that stimulate the anterior pituitary gland

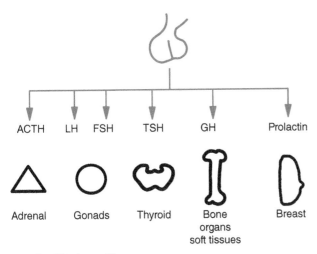

ACTH   LH   FSH   TSH   GH   Prolactin

Adrenal   Gonads   Thyroid   Bone   Breast
                              organs
                              soft tissues

Anterior Pituitary Hormones

to produce its hormones. The hypothalamus makes a hormone that stimulates production of each of the hormones above (except for prolactin, which has no well-defined stimulatory hormone). The hypothalamus also makes inhibitory hormones for some of the anterior pituitary hormones above. The hypothalamic hormones and their actions include:

TRH (thyrotropin-releasing hormone)—stimulates TSH secretion
GHRH (growth hormone-releasing hormone)—stimulates GH secretion
GnRH (gonadotropin-releasing hormone)—stimulates FSH and LH secretion
CRH (corticotropin-releasing hormone)—stimulates ACTH secretion
Dopamine—inhibits prolactin secretion
Somatostatin—inhibits GH and TSH secretion.

Traditionally, it has been felt that prolactin had no well-defined stimulatory hormone, only an inhibitory one (dopamine). Yet, TRH does stimulate prolactin production to a degree. Since the control of prolactin is primarily inhibitory, disorders that disrupt the pituitary stalk (e.g., suprasellar tumors) can cause a mild elevation of prolactin by disrupting the inhibitory mechanism.

The posterior lobe can be envisioned simply as an extension of the hypothalamus; the second class of hypothalamic hormones are those that are secreted by the posterior pituitary gland. These include the antidiuretic hormone (ADH), important in the body's conservation of water. The other, oxytocin, is a nine-amino acid peptide that acts on mammary ducts to facilitate milk letdown during nursing and aids contraction of uterine muscle during childbirth. Oxytocin deficiency causes difficulty with nursing because of impaired milk ejection but is not associated with decreased fertility or delivery.

Oxytocin traditionally has been felt to be of no clinical significance in men, or play a role in women other than in childbirth. Recent research on oxytocin, however, has suggested several other neurobiochemical roles, such as enhancing social interaction. It has been postulated that some individuals with impairment of social interaction (e.g., autism and autism spectrum disorders) may have deficiencies in oxytocin production, and it is being explored as an investigational therapy.

GROWTH HORMONE

When many people think of the pituitary, they think of growth hormone and its obvious disorders, such as pituitary gigantism and dwarfism. Growth hormone is not essential to life in the adult, but is necessary for normal growth and development in childhood and adolescence. It has a direct effect on certain tissues, such as increasing protein synthesis and fatty acid release. It is, in fact, a "stress" hormone and increases during times of increased metabolic demands. Its most striking effects, however, are those on bone and cartilage, where it promotes linear growth. This is not a direct effect of GH, but is mediated through a substance called insulin-like growth factor I (IGF-I); an older name for this molecule is somatomedin C. It is called IGF because it has many effects that are similar to insulin. GH stimulates the liver to produce IGF-I, which then stimulates bone and cartilage to grow. (As we will learn in the reproductive endocrinology lecture, sex steroids (primarily estradiol) are also necessary for normal bone growth; proper secretion of both sex steroids and GH are necessary for achieving normal adult stature and proportions.)

Like many pituitary hormones, GH is secreted in a cyclical manner, with peak levels occurring during sleep. Many factors increase or decrease its secretion. Growth hormone is a stress hormone, so stressors such as exercise increase its concentration. GH tends to promote glucose release, and low blood glucose (hypoglycemia) also is a stimulus for its secretion. In contrast, high blood glucose (hyperglycemia) inhibits its release.

Now is a good time to talk about normal growth and development. For most people, growth is normal and there are no concerns. For others, however, growth is abnormal and we need to distinguish abnormal from normal growth and development. One way is by constructing a growth curve. This is a simple graph made by plotting height versus age. These are usually plotted on graph paper with normal standards for boys and girls. The middle line represents the 50th percentile; the upper and lower lines, the 95th and 5th percentiles, respectively.

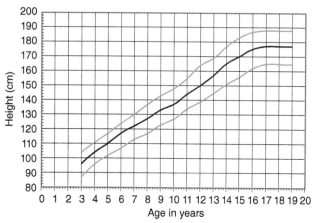

Normal Growth Chart for Boys

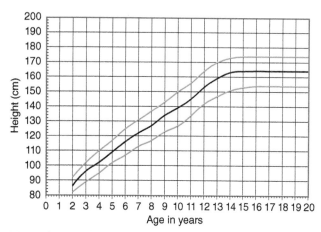

Normal Growth Chart for Girls

Although these curves give us some useful information, more information is learned by constructing a growth velocity curve. This is a little bit more complex than a simple growth curve. In the growth velocity curve, we must first determine the rate of growth at each growth point, plotting against age. For example, if a child grew from 140 to 144 cm in 6 months, the rate of growth would be 4 cm in 6 months or 8 cm/year. The growth rate is highest during infancy, falls off steadily, and then increases again at puberty (the "growth spurt"). As final adult height is attained, the growth velocity obviously falls to zero.

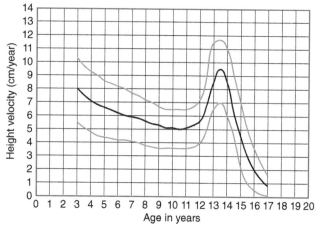

Growth Velocity Chart for Boys

A common question is how to estimate how tall a child will be. This is not always possible to estimate exactly, since many factors play into the final height. Because height is normally distributed, any set of given parents may have children that are either taller or shorter than they are.

Short stature and growth hormone deficiency

One common growth-related complaint is short stature. Our society tends to place emphasis on height and it is natural that some people want to be tall. Height, like weight, intelligence, and many other parameters, is normally distributed; it stands to reason that a small percentage of patients will fall at the lower end, just as a few will fall at the higher end. The challenging goal is to distinguish normal from pathological short stature. The most common cause of short stature is constitutional short stature, which is just a variation from normal for the population. It stands to reason that short parents tend to produce short children. When we look at the growth curves for patients with constitutional short stature, they normally stay at the same percentile throughout their entire growth. For example, a boy who is at the fifth percentile when he is 4 years old will, most likely, be at (or close to) the fifth percentile when he is 12 years old, unless there is a pathological problem. Crossing broad percentiles can raise a red flag for a pathological condition.

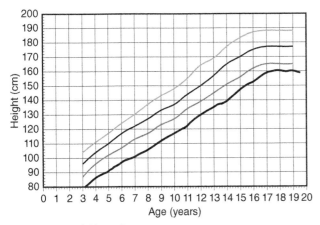

Constitutional Short Stature

What are some pathological causes of short stature? Patients with growth hormone deficiency certainly will have short stature. This is a type of short stature that is proportional (i.e., he or she has normal bodily proportions, but is smaller than normal). Mothers that use drugs or have intrauterine infections (such as rubella) may have children with short stature. Another form of short stature occurs in children who are deprived of attention and affection. This is called psychosocial dwarfism and may be reversible if the child is removed from the dysfunctional environment. Children with severe, chronic medical conditions (e.g., renal failure) may develop short stature. Drugs that inhibit growth (e.g., glucocorticoids) may cause short stature if given in childhood.

Some types of short stature are not proportional. The most common example is achondroplastic dwarfism. In this condition, the face, hands, feet, face, and trunk are normal in size, but the limbs are disproportionately short. The average height of adult men is 52 in. (131 cm); adult women average 49 in. (124 cm). It occurs in 1 in 20,000–40,000 newborns and is inherited in an autosomal dominant fashion as a defect in the FGFR3 (fibroblast growth factor receptor 3) gene. About 80% of achondroplastic patients have normal-sized parents, and a new mutation in FGFR3 has been inherited; the remainder of patients inherited it from one or two affected parents. There is no effective treatment for this disorder.

Growth hormone deficiency is treated with injections of GH. It must usually be given daily, although a depot GH preparation is available. Years ago, GH was scarce, as it had to be procured from cadaver pituitary glands. Fortunately, growth hormone can now be manufactured using genetic engineering technology, ensuring a limitless supply of growth hormone. However, it still is very expensive to produce, and treatment may cost $40,000

per year or more. It is, therefore, important to properly identify individuals who are legitimate candidates for this therapy.

Tall stature and GH excess

Tall stature is generally not a cause for concern because society traditionally (right or wrong) views it as desirable. As with short stature, the most common cause of tall stature is constitutional tall stature occurring in the children of tall parents.

Pathologic causes of tall stature are rare. Gigantism occurs when excess growth hormone is present during childhood or puberty. This results in accelerated bone growth and excessive tall stature. These patients eventually develop disfigurement because of the effects of growth hormone on the face, hands, and feet. The tallest giant on record, Robert Wadlow, was 8 ft 11 in. tall (272 cm) and weighed 490 lb (220 kg) at the time of his death at age 22. Excess growth hormone has many adverse effects on the body, and most giants have a decreased life expectancy.

The average adult height in the United States is 5 ft 9.3 in. (69.3 in. or 176 cm) for men and 5 ft 3.8 in. (63.8 in. or 162 cm) for women. If you watch a professional basketball game, you might wonder how many of these men and women have gigantism, since the average height of male and female professional basketball players is 6 ft 8 in. (80 in. or 203 cm) and 6 ft 0 in. (72 in. or 183 cm), respectively (many players are much taller). You might be surprised to learn that these men and women simply have constitutional tall stature and have no endocrine or genetic abnormality (other than probably having tall parents). If you were to measure the growth hormone levels of a professional basketball player and compare those to same-gender persons with constitutional short stature, you would find comparable levels. There simply are genetic differences in the expression of height that are independent of growth hormone levels. While you might think that giants would be great football or basketball players, wrestlers, and so on, they typically are very poor athletes. Despite their large bulk and muscle mass, their muscles are often weaker than normal and they are prone to develop problems with degenerative arthritis and cardiac disease, often leading to a decreased lifespan.

For a patient to develop gigantism, the growth hormone excess obviously has to occur before the patient has finished growing. A more common disease occurs when growth hormone excess begins in adulthood. This is called acromegaly (from the Greek words *akros*, "extremities," and megalos, "large") is so named because of the enlargement of the face, hands, and feet in these patients. Since these patients are adults when the growth hormone excess starts, the long bones cannot grow further, so that their height remains the same. They do, however, become disfigured, because of the effects of GH on the hands, face, and feet. Acromegaly also may result in enlargement of organs such as the heart, which can lead to cardiac disease and even death. In addition, growth hormone in large concentrations may cause diabetes.

This last complication might seem counterintuitive, since we discussed that growth hormone causes the production of IGF-I by the liver. So why does not GH excess improve glucose metabolism? Although IGF-I does have some insulin-like actions, the anti-insulin effects of excess growth hormone far outweigh this effect of IGF-I, and glucose intolerance results. Hypertension and cardiomyopathy also may result. Patients with acromegaly often develop arthritis and visual field defects due to compression of the optic nerve by the large pituitary tumors.

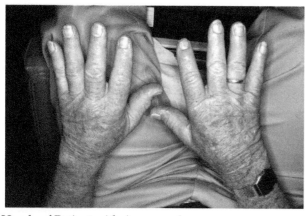

Hands of Patient with Acromegaly

As we have discussed, random measurement of pituitary hormones is often not very useful. When we suspect endocrine excess, we typically do a suppressive study. A natural inhibitor of growth hormone secretion is hyperglycemia, so we commonly perform what is called a glucose tolerance test to evaluate growth hormone excess. Growth hormone is measured before and after the ingestion of a glucose-containing drink (100 g). In normal patients, GH suppresses below a certain level (<2 ng/mL). Patients with either acromegaly or gigantism do not suppress, thus confirming the diagnosis. IGF-I levels are also elevated in acromegaly and/or gigantism.

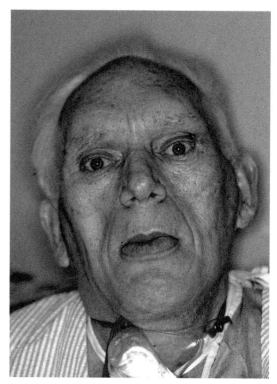

Facial Features of Patient with Acromegaly

Growth hormone-secreting tumors can be treated in several ways. One way is to perform surgery and remove the tumor. Smaller tumors can be removed by a trans-sphenoidal approach (through the roof of the mouth). Larger tumors must be removed via a transfrontal approach (through the forehead).

Remember that a natural inhibitor of growth hormone secretion is the hypothalamic hormone somatostatin. Synthetic hormones such as lanreotide and octreotide are long-acting analogs of somatostatin and in fact inhibit growth hormone-secreting tumors. These medications are given by injection and work well, although in most cases it is an adjunct to surgery. Pegvisomant is a GH receptor antagonist that may be useful in refractory cases (but, unlike somatostatin analogs, it does not directly treat the cause by shrinking the tumor). In severe cases not responsive to either surgery or medication, radiation therapy is used to destroy the tumor.

PROLACTIN

We will next discuss prolactin because it is related to growth hormone—both are derived from a similar precursor and produced by the same cell type. The similarity ends there, however, as they have vastly different physiological functions. The function of prolactin is to stimulate proliferation of lactation (mammary) glands, which results in milk production after birth of an infant. During pregnancy, the increased estrogen levels result in increased prolactin secretion and ductal proliferation in the breast. In the normal postpartum period, lactation results. Another consequence of hyperprolactinemia is decreased gonadotropin secretion. Prolactin levels are typically very high after parturition, and this in fact prevents another pregnancy from occurring until the infant has been weaned from breast milk. This might not be very important today, but it was essential in more primitive times when reliable methods of birth control were not available. It is detrimental for females of any species to be continuously pregnant, so prolactin plays a secondary role in mammals by preventing the family from becoming excessively large. Men do not really need prolactin, and no clinical syndrome results from its deficiency in males.

It should go without saying that pregnancy should be excluded in any woman of reproductive age with amenorrhea. Not doing a simple pregnancy test in such patients can lead to an expensive evaluation of a normal process. Common things are common!

Thus far we have limited our discussion to physiologic prolactin secretion. What happens when prolactin is pathologically secreted? Let us recall what prolactin does. When prolactin is secreted in excess, it suppresses the gonadotropins (LH and FSH), which then results in decreased gonadal function. As mentioned above, this results in amenorrhea (lack of menses) in women. Prolactin excess in men results in hypogonadism and infertility. Unlike in women, however, there is no normal physiologic mechanism that results in hyperprolactinemia in men. Women with excess prolactin may lactate. After childbirth this is obviously desirable. When this occurs otherwise it is called galactorrhea (galactose is the carbohydrate found in milk). Men only rarely have galactorrhea because they lack the high estrogen levels needed for milk production. The most common cause of pathologic prolactin secretion is a prolactin-secreting pituitary tumor, which is called a prolactinoma.

Fortunately, we have an effective way to medically manage these pituitary tumors. Since dopamine is a normal antagonist of prolactin, we may administer a synthetic analog of dopamine that inhibits prolactin secretion. The oldest such drug is bromocriptine, which reduces prolactin levels to normal in many cases. Cabergoline is a long-acting dopamine agonist that can be given once or twice weekly. Once prolactin levels have normalized, the adverse clinical effects of hyperprolactinemia disappear. Very large tumors not responsive to medical therapy ("aggressive" prolactinomas) may require treatment with either surgery or radiation therapy. Fortunately, these nonmedical therapies are necessary only in a minority of cases.

Many medications can cause hyperprolactinemia. These include many commonly used antidepressants and other drugs for psychiatric disorders.

Another common condition that can result in hyperprolactinemia is primary hypothyroidism. In this disorder, the thyroid itself is damaged and cannot respond to normal TSH stimulation. TSH is then produced in large amounts in response to increased thyrotropin-releasing hormone (TRH) secretion from the hypothalamus. TRH appears to increase prolactin as well as TSH secretion. This may occur to such a degree that significant hyperprolactinemia and its consequences (galactorrhea and hypogonadism) may result. Hypothyroidism should therefore be excluded in all patients with hyperprolactinemia. Prolactin levels return to normal after treatment of the hypothyroidism.

Nonpathologic hyperprolactinemia

Other than pregnancy, there is a common cause of hyperprolactinemia called macroprolactinemia. Circulating prolactin in serum is not glycosylated and is 23 kD in size; in some cases, however, glycosylated prolactin (which circulates in aggregates), accounts for most of the prolactin, up to 170 kD in size. This form of prolactin is called "big" or "macro" prolactin. This "macroprolactin" of aggregated glycosylated molecules (and sometimes antibodies) is biologically inert and causes hyperprolactinemia, since the kidney inefficiently clears this larger form. This is a benign condition (as this compound is nonfunctional) and the presence of macroprolactin can be detected by special laboratory methods. This condition needs to be considered when asymptomatic patients present with hyperprolactinemia. Failure to recognize this can result in unnecessary and costly imaging, treatment, and so on.

PITUITARY TUMORS

Let us now shift our focus to pituitary tumors in general. Pituitary tumors may be classified as microadenomas (<1 cm in diameter) or macroadenomas (≥1 cm in diameter).

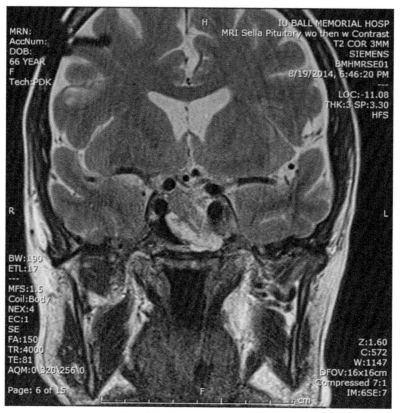

MRI of Pituitary Macroadenoma

Some pituitary tumors produce hormones, such as growth hormone or prolactin. Other tumors are nonfunctional (i.e., they do not make any hormones). These nonfunctional or nonsecretory pituitary tumors account for approximately 10% of all pituitary tumors; most often these cells are of gonadotroph origin (but do not make functional hormones). These "incidental tumors" may be found on a CT (computed tomogram) or an MRI scan done for another reason (later, we will discuss incidental thyroid and adrenal masses, which are frequently encountered as well). Although nonfunctional tumors do not produce hormone excess syndromes, they may still cause damage and endocrine deficiency because of their size and destruction of adjacent cells.

Pituitary tumors may cause headache and/or visual field defects and potentially hypopituitarism. The pituitary lies right above the optic chiasm (where the optic nerves cross on the way to the eyes). Because nonfunctional tumors are non-hormone-secreting, they do not respond to specific medical treatment as some that are hormone-secreting (e.g., prolactinomas, GH tumors, etc.) do. Large tumors causing mass-effect problems may need to be reduced surgically or with radiotherapy.

HYPOPITUITARISM

Hypopituitarism is a condition resulting from the deficiency of one or more pituitary hormones; panhypopituitarism is the deficiency of all pituitary hormones. The most common cause is destruction of the gland by a pituitary tumor. Surgery and irradiation of the pituitary also commonly cause hypopituitarism. Severe head trauma can damage the pituitary stalk. Tumors that destroy the hypothalamus result in hypothalamic hormone deficiency and hypopituitarism. This is called "tertiary" hormone deficiency. Hypopituitarism can also be the result of genetic defects (e.g., defects in the PROP1 or POUF1 genes), or other conditions (e.g., cranial radiation for malignancies of childhood, tumor such as craniopharyngiomas, etc.).

What are the clinical consequences of panhypopituitarism? Some of these hormones are necessary for life. The body cannot survive without thyroid hormone and adrenocortical hormones; without the trophic hormones TSH and ACTH, death occurs. Fortunately, thyroid hormone (thyroxine) and cortisol (hydrocortisone) are inexpensive and easily absorbed orally. Gonadotropin

(LH and FSH) deficiency, although not life threatening, results in hypogonadism and infertility. Deficiency of growth hormone in childhood results in an adult with proportional short stature. Growth hormone deficiency in adults has no devastating consequences, although recent research suggests that growth hormone plays an essential role in maintaining normal bone and muscle metabolism. Adults who lack growth hormone tend to become less muscular and have a greater proportion of fat. Therefore, some adults with GH deficiency are now treated. Prolactin deficiency has no clinical consequences except for the lack of postpartum lactation. This is hardly life threatening in industrialized countries, as commercial infant formulas are readily available (although the other benefits of human milk to the infant are lost). One interesting cause of panhypopituitarism occurs in the postpartum period in women who experience severe postpartum hemorrhage. This condition, called Sheehan's syndrome, results in pituitary damage and hypopituitarism, including the inability to lactate. Hormone replacement is necessary in these women.

Another rare condition that can occur in late-gestation or postpartum women is lymphocytic hypophysitis. This is an autoimmune inflammation of the pituitary that can result in panhypopituitarism.

Pituitary (secondary) hypothyroidism is treated by administration of synthetic thyroid hormone (levothyroxine). This is the same treatment as for primary hypothyroidism (as administration of recombinant TSH would be both impractical (injection) and horribly expensive); however, we monitor the treatment differently. As we will learn later in the thyroid lecture, we often monitor primary hypothyroidism treatment by measuring the trophic hormone (serum TSH), and the goal is to maintain it within the normal range (this is often more sensitive than measuring the peripheral level, which has a broad "normal" range); TSH increases exponentially out of its normal range in primary hypothyroidism, making it a sensitive test. TSH, however is *not* a reliable indicator of thyroid hormone status in secondary (or tertiary) hypothyroidism, since it is, obviously, already deficient. Instead of monitoring TSH, we must then measure peripheral hormone (T4 or T3) levels.

Treatment of hypogonadism involves replacement of sex steroids. In women, estrogen is easily replaced orally, which is the preferred method of administration; it may also be administered as a transdermal patch. Estrogen should be given to all women of premenopausal age who do not have contraindications (e.g., breast carcinoma,

active thromboembolic disease). Estrogen administration in postmenopausal women is controversial and will be discussed in the calcium and reproductive endocrinology lectures.

Testosterone is metabolized rapidly by the liver and is therefore not useful as an oral medication. It may be administered by intramuscular injection, transdermal patch, or gel, or by other methods (new preparations have been developed with delivery via nasal or buccal administration).

One interesting difference between primary and secondary (pituitary) hypogonadism is that, in theory, fertility may be restored in the latter. Fertility is generally impossible in primary hypogonadism since the gonad is permanently damaged. With secondary hypogonadism, however, the gonad is structurally intact but does not work properly because of inadequate stimulation. We can, therefore, administer the gonadotropins themselves, which stimulate the gonads to work properly. This is much easier to accomplish in men than in women, because of the complexity of the female reproductive cycle.

Pituitary apoplexy is a serious endocrine emergency. This is caused by spontaneous hemorrhage into the pituitary, which results in pituitary damage and hypopituitarism. These patients usually present with severe headache, blurred vision, and confusion. This constitutes an emergency and requires prompt treatment with glucocorticoids and thyroid hormone (since these hormones are necessary for life).

POSTERIOR PITUITARY

Antidiuretic hormone

The posterior pituitary hormones, ADH and oxytocin, are produced in the supraoptic and paraventricular nuclei of the hypothalamus and travel to the posterior pituitary by means of nerve fibers. ADH (arginine vasopressin) is of great importance in humans; its major function is to help the body regulate water metabolism. Increased ADH levels increase water reabsorption by the kidney; decreased ADH levels result in increased water loss through the kidneys. This mechanism can be advantageous in several circumstances. Imagine a person who is running a summer marathon. This person may become very dehydrated, and ADH levels increase in an effort to hold on to whatever water is present in the body.

In contrast, visualize a person who drank too much water. ADH levels decrease so that the body can excrete this excess water, restoring water balance to normal. If this does not happen, he or she may become water intoxicated, which can lead to problems such as hyponatremia (low sodium levels) and confusion.

Diabetes insipidus

Diabetes insipidus (DI) is a disorder in which ADH is either deficient or does not have appropriate action. (It is not related to diabetes mellitus, which is a disorder of glucose metabolism that we will discuss later.) These patients cannot hold on to appropriate amounts of water and therefore urinate quite frequently, sometimes passing over 10 liters of urine per day. They must constantly drink water to replace the amount that is lost in the urine, and this can lead to significant lifestyle disruptions. Patients with diabetes insipidus typically keep water at the bedside so they have something to drink when they wake up, and they are unable to take any long trips without having to stop at the restroom quite often. They also have all the restroom locations at the local shopping malls (and other frequently visited places) memorized. If your patient with untreated diabetes insipidus must wait very long in your office, you will probably see him or her make several trips to the drinking fountain and the bathroom, with the ubiquitous large drink always at hand.

There are two types of DI. The first results from a deficiency of ADH, and is called central or neurogenic DI. This often results from some type of pituitary or hypothalamic damage secondary to trauma or surgery. It also may present for no apparent reason (idiopathic). The second type of diabetes insipidus is called nephrogenic DI and is a hormone resistance syndrome rather than a deficiency syndrome. This means that adequate amounts of ADH are produced, but the kidney is unresponsive to it. This condition results from a variety of renal disorders, and is frequently seen in patients on lithium therapy for psychiatric disorders.

Patients with diabetes insipidus can survive as long as they have free access to water and have an intact thirst mechanism. If the patient is denied free access to water (e.g., if they are hospitalized for an acute illness) they may become dehydrated. This type of lifestyle however is very disruptive, and therapy is recommended to most patients with diabetes insipidus. Central diabetes insipidus is easily treated with the synthetic ADH derivative desmopressin. ADH itself is typically not used because it is degraded very rapidly and has other effects such as increasing blood pressure (hence the name vasopressin). Desmopressin is very long lasting and is devoid of these other effects which are not desired. Desmopressin may be given subcutaneously, as a nasal spray, or as oral tablets, yet this therapy is not without potential risk: patients without an intact thirst mechanism may develop problems if they drink too little water (they become dehydrated) or if they drink too much water (becoming water intoxicated).

There are several medications that augment the action of ADH. These medications are useful in patients who make a little bit of ADH but are ineffective in those who do not make ADH at all. These medications include chlorpropamide (an oral agent also used for type 2 diabetes), carbamazepine (an anticonvulsant), and clofibrate (a lipid-lowering medication). They are of historical interest and are seldom used today.

Nephrogenic diabetes insipidus is less easily treated. Since the patient already makes adequate amounts of ADH, giving extra ADH does not help since they are resistant to it. Some diuretics (e.g., amiloride), surprisingly, actually enhance free water absorption and are useful in many patients.

There are conditions other than DI that can result in polyuria and polydipsia. The most significant to exclude is diabetes mellitus. Another relatively common cause is psychogenic polydipsia (compulsive water drinking). This is a condition in which the patient consumes too much water (often greater than 10 gal/day). Many of these patients have underlying psychiatric problems and often take medications that cause dry mouth, thus prompting them to drink too much water. Psychogenic polydipsia is treated by restricting water intake and treating the underlying behavioral disorder.

SIADH

Bad things can also occur when the body has too much ADH (or most other hormones, for that matter); excess ADH results in a disorder exactly the opposite of diabetes insipidus, called the syndrome of inappropriate antidiuretic hormone (SIADH). These patients present with hyponatremia (low sodium levels), are by definition euvolemic (i.e., not fluid overloaded from renal or cardiac failure) and have no other endocrine abnormality (hypothyroidism and adrenal insufficiency can cause hyponatremia). Hyponatremia in SIADH may cause confusion, coma, seizures, and even death in severe cases.

A common cause of SIADH is malignancy. Certain tumors such as small cell lung carcinoma commonly make neuroendocrine peptides such as ADH. Patients with head trauma may experience release of ADH from the hypothalamus. SIADH may also be caused by nonmalignant lung conditions (e.g., pneumonia). Several medications can cause SIADH. Patients taking chlorpropamide, carbamazepine, or clofibrate (all of which potentiate ADH action and thus can be used in the treatment of partial central diabetes insipidus) may develop SIADH. Opioid analgesics such as morphine may potentiate ADH action and result in hyponatremia. At times, no cause for the SIADH can be found (idiopathic). SIADH may be distinguished from primary polydipsia (water intoxication) since ADH levels are inappropriately high in the former, and suppressed in the latter. It is important to exclude other endocrine causes of hyponatremia (e.g., adrenal insufficiency) before a diagnosis of SIADH is entertained.

The first way to treat SIADH is to treat any underlying condition such as malignancy. The next step is generally to restrict the patient's fluids. If this is unsuccessful, a medication called demeclocycline may be used. This negates the effect of ADH on the kidney and restores normal function. Two vasopressin receptor antagonists (conivaptan and tolvaptan) are also useful in cases of severe hyponatremia due to SIADH.

Oxytocin

Oxytocin stimulates milk ejection from mammary glands and therefore plays a vital role in lactation. It also stimulates uterine contraction and aids in delivery of the fetus at parturition. Labor can occur in the absence of oxytocin, but it proceeds more slowly. Oxytocin is often given during labor to help with uterine contractions and to decrease postpartum bleeding. Deficiency of oxytocin has classically been felt to have clinical consequences in women who are not giving birth or lactating; recent research into the neurobiochemical roles of oxytocin discussed earlier may disprove this theory.

REVIEW QUESTIONS

1. You are asked to evaluate a 16-year-old man for tall stature. He stands 6 ft 7 in. (201 cm) and weighs 240 lb (108 kg). Father is 5 ft 7 in. and mother is 5 ft 4 in.. Physical examination is unremarkable except for large size. Puberty occurred at age 13; he has normal secondary sexual development and potency. Arm span equals height. Growth hormone level drawn 60 min after a 100 g glucose load is 32.1 ng/mL (normal response: <3 ng/mL). Serum prolactin is normal.

   a. What do you think the diagnosis is?

   b. How would you evaluate this patient further?

   c. What are the treatment options?

   d. What are the consequences of no or inadequate treatment?

   (a) The differential diagnosis is constitutional tall stature versus gigantism. His target height is only 68 in., and an 11 in. differential is unusual. He also has a grossly abnormal response to glucose suppression, confirming a diagnosis of growth hormone excess.

   (b) An IGF-I level would be useful. GH excess is usually caused by pituitary tumors, so MRI imaging is mandatory. Evaluation of other hormones should be performed as well.

   (c) The mainstay of treatment is resection of the pituitary tumor. Adjunct therapy can include long-acting somatostatin analogs such as octreotide or lanreotide; the GH receptor antagonist pegvisomant may be useful in some cases (unlike somatostatin analogs; however, pegvisomant only blocks the effect of GH and does not shrink tumor size). Radiotherapy/gamma knife therapy may be useful in some cases.

   (d) Without treatment, he may continue to grow further. The deleterious effects of continued organ involvement cannot be reversed, and he is at risk for cardiomyopathy. Giants and patients with acromegaly are much more prone to have degenerative joint disease at an early age.

2. A 47-year-old woman presents to the emergency department with severe headache, diplopia, nausea, and vomiting. She is hypotensive and laboratory studies are remarkable for hyponatremia and low random serum cortisol. MRI of the head demonstrates a 1.5 cm pituitary tumor with acute hemorrhage. In addition to consulting the neurosurgeon on call, what would your next step in management be?

   a. Admission and promptly starting intravenous fluids and hydrocortisone, adding levothyroxine the next day

b. Admission and promptly starting intravenous fluids and levothyroxine, adding hydrocortisone the next day

c. Admission and promptly starting intravenous fluids, hydrocortisone, levothyroxine, and estrogen

d. Admission and performing an ACTH stimulation test and starting hydrocortisone the next day if abnormal

(a) This is a classic presentation of pituitary apoplexy, a true endocrine emergency. In addition to neurosurgical consultation and surgical decompression of the tumor, she should receive stress doses of glucocorticoids, with thyroid hormone added later. Starting levothyroxine before glucocorticoids would be hazardous and would potentially worsen the situation. Estrogen (c) is not necessary in emergency management of hypopituitarism. Waiting for laboratory results (d) could have catastrophic consequences; hypotension with a low random cortisol level would be considered sufficient "stress" to result in an elevated serum cortisol in a normal person.

3. A 21-year-old college student presents with a 2-month history of weight gain, mild nausea, and amenorrhea. She takes no medications. Physical examination is unremarkable. The student health center checked the serum prolactin level, which is three times normal. Examination is remarkable for fullness in the thyroid. The next best test to order to confirm the most likely diagnosis is:

a. Pituitary MRI

b. Serum TSH

c. Progestational challenge

d. Serum pregnancy test

(d) Common things are common, and the most likely etiology of amenorrhea, weight gain, and hyperprolactinemia in a young woman is pregnancy. MRI (a) is obviously not warranted. She does have a small goiter, but this is common in pregnancy; checking TSH to rule out primary hypothyroidism as the cause of hyperprolactinemia would be reasonable if pregnancy is ruled out. Progestational challenge (c) would be harmful to the fetus if pregnancy is present.

LECTURE 3 The Thyroid

REVIEW

Let us now review what we learned in the last lecture. We learned about the "quarterback" of our team—the pituitary and hypothalamus, which essentially function together as 1 unit called the hypothalamic–pituitary axis (HPA).

The pituitary is a small gland that is divided into the anterior and posterior lobes. The anterior pituitary makes hormones such as ACTH, growth hormone (GH), prolactin, thyroid-stimulating hormone (TSH), and the gonadotropins (LH and FSH), which control specific glands. The posterior pituitary is actually an extension of the brain. Hormones secreted by this organ include antidiuretic hormone (ADH or arginine vasopressin) and oxytocin.

Growth hormone (GH) is not essential for life in the adult, but is necessary for normal growth in children and adolescents. It has a direct effect on some tissues, but its main effects are mediated by a molecule called insulin-like growth factor I (IGF-I), which is made in the liver. Deficiency of growth hormone results in short stature in children, and may be treated with synthetic growth hormone. Growth hormone therapy has also been shown to provide benefits for adults with GH deficiency. Short stature is a common presenting complaint to any physician who sees children. Most children with short stature have constitutional short stature (e.g., a child of short parents).

Like short stature, most cases of tall stature have no pathologic cause—the most common cause is constitutional tall stature. Growth hormone excess in childhood results in gigantism. Many patients with gigantism are seven feet tall or more (although many people seven feet tall are not giants; they are merely on the extremes of human stature). Growth hormone excess in adults results in a condition called acromegaly, which causes disfigurement with increased growth of the facial bones, hands, and feet. Growth hormone excess is usually caused by a pituitary tumor.

The hormone prolactin is necessary for normal lactation in women, and has other functions. It plays a less significant role in men, but prolactin appears to enhance luteinizing hormone receptors in Leydig cells, resulting in testosterone secretion, which assists in spermatogenesis. Increased prolactin (hyperprolactinemia) may result from a variety of causes. A common cause is a pituitary tumor, although medications may cause hyperprolactinemia. Galactorrhea is the presence of milk in the absence of pregnancy and is a common presenting complaint of hyperprolactinemia in women. Hypogonadism may occur in both men and women with hyperprolactinemia.

Pituitary tumors may produce hormones or may be nonfunctional. Tumors that are very large may cause endocrine effects by destroying the pituitary itself, causing hypopituitarism. Panhypopituitarism is the deficiency of all pituitary hormones. Other causes of hypopituitarism include pituitary surgery and irradiation. Hypothalamic destruction results in hypopituitarism. Panhypopituitarism may result in death due to deficiency of ACTH and TSH, but this may be treated by the administration of synthetic corticosteroids and thyroid hormone. Deficiencies of the other hormones do not result in death but may result in significant morbidity.

ADH (arginine vasopressin) is the major hormone of the posterior pituitary. It is important in regulating the body's fluid balance. ADH increases water retention by the kidney. Decreased levels therefore result in increased water loss. Central or neurogenic diabetes insipidus (DI) is a condition in which the pituitary makes too little ADH. These patients cannot hold onto water and have incessant thirst and urination. This condition is easily treated by administration of ADH. Another cause of diabetes insipidus occurs when the body is resistant to ADH. This condition is less easily treated. Persons with DI must be distinguished from those with psychogenic polydipsia (water intoxication), who simply drink too much water.

The opposite of diabetes insipidus is syndrome of inappropriate antidiuretic hormone (SIADH). This syndrome is most commonly caused by tumors that make ADH, but may also be caused by other conditions or medications. These patients have too much water and may develop severe electrolyte disturbances. Restricting water intake and administering drugs that inhibit the action of ADH can treat this condition.

THE THYROID

The largest endocrine organ is the thyroid. It has two lobes, an isthmus (middle) and a small embryonic remnant, the pyramidal lobe. The normal thyroid weighs about 20 g, but may become enlarged to many times this size in disease states.

The thyroid is important for many reasons. Thyroid hormones are necessary for life, and have a variety of functions. They increase the body's metabolism, resulting in increased oxygen consumption, heart contractility, intestinal motility, bone remodeling, and degradation of many substances (e.g., cholesterol, medications, other hormones). In our analogy of the endocrine system as a football team, the thyroid is like the offensive linemen who help the other players catch passes and move downfield. Without enough thyroid hormone, the body basically "slows down" and becomes sluggish (kind of like playing a video in slow motion). Too much thyroid hormone results in a stimulated individual (like playing a video too fast).

THYROID HORMONES

The major molecule made by the thyroid is the hormone 3,5,3′,5′-tetraiodothyronine or thyroxine (T4). T4 is made from two modified tyrosine molecules hooked together with four iodine atoms attached (hence the name T4). T4 is highly protein bound, and for a hormone has a very long serum half-life (1 week). In the blood, T4 loses one iodine atom, and the hormone triiodothyronine or T3 is formed (the thyroid does make some T3, but most results from peripheral deiodination). This new hormone is much more potent than T4. You might ask, then: why

does not the thyroid just make T3 instead of T4? The reason is that T4 lasts much longer in the blood than T3 (half-life of approximately 7 days vs 1 day). T4 therefore serves as a "storage reservoir" for later conversion to T3.

3,5,3′,5-L-Tetraiodothyronine (thyroxine, T4)

3,5,3′-L-Triiodothyronine (T3)

T4 and T3

The stimulus for thyroid hormone secretion is TSH, produced by the pituitary gland. (TSH is not properly called a "thyroid hormone" because it is a trophic glycoprotein hormone made in the pituitary gland.)

The functional unit of the thyroid where thyroid hormones are synthesized is the follicle, which is under strict control by TSH. Thyroid hormone synthesis starts when iodine atoms are brought into the follicular cell by means of a process called trapping. Since the iodine content inside the follicle is much greater than outside the follicle, this requires active transport (i.e., against a concentration gradient). Once the iodine atoms are inside the thyroid follicle, they are activated to an oxidized state by thyroid peroxidase (TPO). While this is going on, the protein thyroglobulin is being synthesized in the thyroid follicle and tyrosine residues are attached to these molecules. After this backbone is assembled, the activated iodine molecules are incorporated into the thyroglobulin molecule by a process called organification. After some rearrangement, the result is T4 attached to the thyroglobulin molecule. The resulting T4–thyroglobulin complex is then moved to the proteinaceous substance in the center of the follicle called the colloid where it may be stored for long periods of time. The thyroid is somewhat unique in that it can store its hormone for weeks at a time unlike most other glands, which synthesize their hormone as needed.

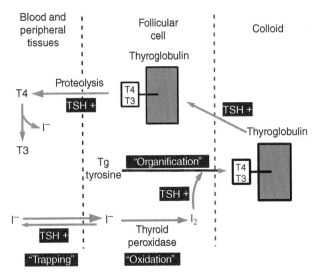
Thyroid Hormone Synthesis

EFFECTS OF THYROID HORMONE

Unlike many hormones that have effects only on certain organs, the thyroid hormones have effects in almost all tissues of the body. A primary role of thyroid hormone is to increase energy expenditure and thermogenesis. Hence, persons with thyroid hormone deficiency complain of cold intolerance.

Protein, carbohydrate, and lipid metabolism are affected by the iodothyronines. Low doses of thyroid hormones promote glycogen synthesis, whereas larger doses stimulate glycogen breakdown. Intestinal absorption of glucose is also accelerated by thyroid hormone. Cholesterol metabolism is depressed in thyroid hormone deficiency, and levels rise in those with hypothyroidism, leading to increased risk of atherosclerosis.

THYROID REGULATION

How is homeostasis maintained? Our "quarterback" (the pituitary gland) plays a major role in regulation of the thyroid gland. When T4 and T3 levels become too low, the pituitary and hypothalamus detect this, and increased TRH and TSH production results. Increased TSH then results in the return of normal T4 levels by increasing synthesis through any mechanisms outlined above. The opposite occurs when T4 levels get too high: TRH and TSH levels diminish, with resultant decreased hormone synthesis and return of levels to normal.

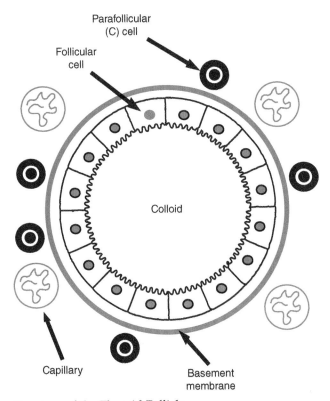
Structure of the Thyroid Follicle

When thyroid hormone is needed, the T4–thyroglobulin complex passes from the colloid into the follicular cell and T4 is cleaved from the complex, yielding T4 molecules that flow into the bloodstream. In the peripheral circulation T4 is then deiodinated to T3, the active hormone (T3 is several times more potent than T4 on a molar basis, but T4 has a much longer half-life).

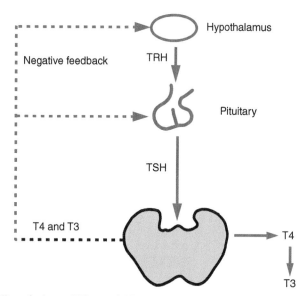

TRH

Hypothalamus

Negative feedback

Pituitary

TSH

T4 and T3

T4

T3

Regulation of Thyroid Hormone Secretion

As we learned from the overview chapter, only the free or unbound portion (about 0.04% of the total hormone for T4) is biologically active (the bound portion is not). The early T4 or T3 assays (still used in many laboratories) measured the total hormone level; in most cases, the difference between measuring the total or free species is not clinically significant. There are, however, some conditions that change the concentration of binding proteins without changing the total level. Measuring the free or unbound portion eliminates these problems and is preferred to measuring total levels.

There are other commonly used tests of thyroid function in addition to the serum hormone assays. A thyroid scan is performed by giving a known amount of radioactive iodine (^{123}I) to the patient in oral form. The patient returns the next day, and a scan image of the thyroid is produced with a large device called a gamma camera. Although the term "gamma camera" sounds ominous, this device is merely a large camera that takes pictures of gamma rays, just as your digital camera takes pictures of visible light.

This procedure yields a low-resolution, two-dimensional picture of the thyroid that can point out structural abnormalities such as thyroid nodules. Another piece of information obtained from this study is the thyroid uptake, which is the fractional amount of radioiodine that has accumulated in the patient's thyroid at 24 h (accounting for the amount that is lost by natural decay, of course). A normal uptake is about 20–35% in the United States. This amount varies depending on iodine

intake in the diet, and is higher in iodine-deficient parts of the world.

Remember this well: radioiodine uptake may or may not correlate with thyroid hormone output. Those with very low uptake values may have hypothyroidism, while those with high values may have hyperthyroidism. This is not always the case, however! Serum biochemistry rather than radioiodine uptake must be used to establish thyroid hormone status before attempting to correlate with an uptake/scan. Radioiodine studies cannot distinguish iodine "trapping" (i.e., active transport into the thyroid epithelial cell) from "organification" (actual incorporation of that iodine into iodothyronine molecules; it is possible to have the former without the latter.

There are two types of radioactive iodine used in nuclear medicine: iodine-123 (^{123}I) and iodine-131 (^{131}I). All isotopes of iodine have the same number of protons ($Z = 53$ for iodine) and hence the same chemical properties, but different neutron (N) and mass (A) numbers (stable iodine is iodine-127). ^{123}I has a very short half-life, emits low energy gamma rays, and is primarily used for thyroid uptake and scan studies.

^{131}I emits high-energy gamma rays plus β particles (electrons) and is not routinely used for scanning, but rather when actual destruction of the thyroid is desired (e.g., in thyroid cancer and hyperthyroidism). Another isotope, iodine-124 (^{124}I) emits positrons and is being studied experimentally as a potential PET imaging tool.

Thyroid ultrasound is another commonly performed procedure. This is noninvasive and exposes the patient to no radiation. Ultrasound gives detailed cross-sections of the thyroid, revealing anatomic structures that cannot be seen with radioiodine scans. While there are some features of ultrasound thyroid images (e.g., ill-defined margins, microcalcifications, hypoechoic pattern) that help distinguish benign from malignant lesions, no imaging procedure can do this with complete certainty.

HYPOTHYROIDISM

We will discuss hypothyroidism first in our thyroid lecture because it is by far the most common thyroid disease and probably the most common endocrine disease (although type 2 diabetes is quickly catching up). Hypothyroidism is a condition in which the thyroid hormone levels are too low. Usually, hypothyroidism is primary in nature (i.e., due to failure of the thyroid gland itself). Less commonly, hypothyroidism may be secondary (due to pituitary failure) or tertiary (due to hypothalamic dysfunction).

The most common cause of primary hypothyroidism in the United States is a disease called Hashimoto's disease or Hashimoto's thyroiditis. Like many endocrine deficiency disorders, it is an autoimmune disease (caused by antithyroid antibodies, usually directed against the peroxidase enzyme important in iodothyronine synthesis), resulting in inefficient hormonogenesis and gland destruction. It is one of the most common autoimmune diseases, and like all autoimmune disorders, seems to occur more frequently in women. Most patients with Hashimoto's thyroiditis have thyroid enlargement (goiter). Another, less common type of primary hypothyroidism is called autoimmune atrophic thyroiditis. In this disorder, TSH-blocking antibodies block the effect of TSH on the thyroid, leading to an atrophic gland.

Other common causes of primary hypothyroidism include thyroidectomy (e.g., for thyroid cancer and obstructive goiter) and ^{131}I ablation for hyperthyroidism. Iodine deficiency is rare in the United States but is still a common cause of hypothyroidism in underdeveloped countries. There are many drugs (e.g., lithium) that can also cause hypothyroidism. Amiodarone (an iodine-containing antiarrhythmic agent) can cause either hypo- or hyperthyroidism; the former is more common in the United States. Amiodarone-induced hyperthyroidism can be especially difficult to treat.

In primary hypothyroidism, the thyroid fails to produce enough thyroid hormone, leading to low T4 and T3 levels. Because the pituitary is still intact, TSH levels rise. The elevated TSH level is the most sensitive indicator of hypothyroidism.

Too little thyroid hormone results in a sluggish individual with decreased energy. He or she often feels cold, complains of dry skin, muscle cramps, slowed mentation and speech, irregular menses (women), and constipation. Patients are able to perform normal activities in most cases. Obesity is not a result of hypothyroidism, contrary to the beliefs of many people (although hypothyroidism can result in modest weight gain). Most adults adapt to hypothyroidism quite well, and the symptoms abate after therapy. In cases of severe hypothyroidism, a condition called myxedema coma results, and has a high mortality rate even with treatment.

Hypothyroidism in young children has more serious consequences. Cretinism is a condition caused by hypothyroidism in very young children and results in short stature and mental retardation. This is really the only endocrine syndrome that results in mental retardation. (This excludes genetic syndromes, for example, Prader–Willi, which can be associated with mental retardation and endocrine deficiency; here, the mental retardation is from the genetic defect, not the hormonal defect.) Fortunately, cretinism is extremely rare today, because mandatory testing for hypothyroidism in neonates is required in the United States and most developed countries. Congenital hypothyroidism is actually fairly common (about 1 in 4,000 live births); thus, prompt recognition and treatment is essential.

Luckily, hypothyroidism is easily and inexpensively treated, as T4 is well absorbed orally. T4 is a small molecule that easily survives the cooking process, so one initial oral treatment of hypothyroidism was to give the patient cooked animal thyroid glands. The next step was to make purer preparations from porcine and bovine thyroid glands (readily available since these animals are consumed for their meat), which are still available today. The preferred treatment today is synthetic levothyroxine, given once per day. Organic molecules come in both "right-handed" (dextro-) and "left-handed" (levo-) forms—almost all such molecules found in living organisms are the left-handed variety. Right-handed molecules (e.g., dextrothyroxine) are not usable by the body. The synthetic T4 is metabolized to T3 in the bloodstream, just like T4 secreted from the thyroid.

Synthetic T4 is preferred to preparations made from animal thyroid glands, because it can be made with greater purity. We could give T3, but this is not ideal because its short half-life requires several doses per day (plus, giving T4 mimics what the body does, for the most part). Current research does not show any benefit in treating patients with both T3 and T4. ("Natural" thyroid products, such as extract from animal thyroids, contain active T3 as well as T4. They have not been proved to be superior to synthetic levothyroxine.)

Since hypothyroidism is common in young women, special attention must be given to those who become pregnant. Thyroid hormone requirements increase by about 30–35% during pregnancy, due to increased blood volume and metabolic demands. While the euthyroid woman can compensate by increasing her thyroid hormone output, the female with hypothyroidism obviously cannot do so. The fetus cannot manufacture its own thyroid hormone until after 12 weeks' gestation, so it is necessary to increase the dosage of thyroid hormone by about 30% immediately once pregnancy is discovered; patients are monitored frequently. Since T4 has a long half-life, this can easily be accomplished by having the patient take two extra T4 tablets weekly (approximately a 30% increase). After delivery, doses revert back to the pre-pregnancy amount.

It must also be remembered that "normal" TSH values are lower in pregnancy than in the nonpregnant woman. The glycoprotein hormone β-hCG (human chorionic gonadotropin) has mild TSH-like effects in the high concentrations seen in pregnancy, so the same amount of TSH is not necessary, resulting in lower levels; this fact should be kept in mind when titrating therapy. Peripheral hormone measurements (free T4) should also be monitored in pregnancy, with the goal of keeping it in the upper normal range.

Treatment of primary hypothyroidism is monitored with routine TSH tests. With adequate treatment, the TSH returns to normal. In secondary hypothyroidism, the hormone levels themselves must be measured, since TSH secretion is already deficient.

Are there any circumstances in which hypothyroidism might actually be beneficial? For patients with severe coronary artery disease, hypothyroidism may be protective. The lowered basal metabolic rate protects the heart from working too hard. To this day there are actually three "approved" indications for therapeutic use of radioiodine (^{131}I). You may be aware of two (hyperthyroidism and thyroid carcinoma), but the third is an archaic one of historical significance: treatment of unstable angina. Remember, 40 or 50 years ago there was no such thing as coronary artery bypass grafting, angioplasty, or other interventional procedures for cardiac patients, nor was medical therapy very advanced (nitroglycerin was the mainstay of therapy). There just was not much available to help these folks with bad heart disease. For selected persons with coronary disease, hypothyroidism was actually induced by giving ^{131}I, which helped prolong their lives. While this indication is archaic, understanding history may help you understand the biological effects of these hormones.

Similarly, treatment of hypothyroidism today in persons with coronary disease can still be risky business; overzealous replacement can precipitate angina or even a myocardial infarction. It is best to try and correct underlying problems, if possible, before starting therapy. If therapy must be started, it should be initiated at the lowest possible dose (e.g., 12.5–25 μg/day of levothyroxine) and titrated upwards very slowly.

HYPERTHYROIDISM AND THYROTOXICOSIS

This is the opposite of hypothyroidism, and is caused by thyroid hormone levels that are too high. The terms hyperthyroidism and thyrotoxicosis actually mean two different things. Thyrotoxicosis refers to excess thyroid hormone from any source (inside or outside the body); hyperthyroidism refers to increased thyroid hormone levels from the body's own thyroid (endogenous). Thyrotoxicosis results in an "accelerated," hyperkinetic individual. Symptoms include weight loss, tachycardia (fast heart rate), increased appetite, tremors, inability to tolerate heat, and diarrhea. At first glance, it might seem beneficial to have all this excess energy and be able to do things much more quickly. Some patients with thyrotoxicosis, in fact, feel this way.

While thought processes may indeed be faster, thyrotoxic persons often make mental errors. An analogy in the computer world is the "overclocking" of a computer microprocessor. Early personal computer users discovered that running a microprocessor at a higher speed resulted in a faster computer without having to pay for a more expensive chip. For example, many users ran their old 300 MHz processors at 450 MHz, to gain extra speed at no cost. The computers indeed were faster, but computational errors and early microprocessor breakdown (due to processor core overheating) were the frequent penalties of such computational misadventures.

To the lay person, another potentially desirable effect of thyrotoxicosis is the ability to lose weight easily. Many patients with thyrotoxicosis find that they can eat anything they want and still keep their weight down; losing weight while eating several thousand kilocalories per day is not uncommon in this setting. At closer inspection, however, this is not such a good thing. The excess thyroid hormone does not burn off only fat but also bone and muscle. Indeed, patients with thyrotoxicosis often have significant muscle weakness and even develop osteoporosis because of the increased bone breakdown. It is much better for the patient to be a little overweight and have normal thyroid hormone levels then be thin and hyperthyroid; it is not a good weight-loss method.

We may define hyperthyroidism (endogenous thyrotoxicosis) as either primary or secondary. Primary refers to the thyroid itself producing too much thyroid hormone without help from the pituitary gland. In primary hyperthyroidism, therefore, TSH levels are low since the pituitary wants nothing to do with this process. T4 and T3 levels are, of course, elevated. Almost all hyperthyroidism is primary in nature and we will focus on this. Secondary hyperthyroidism results from excessive production of TSH by pituitary tumors (or, even more rarely, genetic syndromes of resistance to thyroid hormone), and, as we will discuss later, is extremely uncommon.

Three basic mechanisms can result in thyrotoxicosis with low TSH. First, the thyroid may synthesize too much thyroid hormone. Second, the thyroid can "leak" large amounts of hormone that has already been made and is in storage (remember that the colloid is a vast reservoir of stored thyroid hormone unlike most endocrine organs that do not have a substantial storage of their hormones). Finally, a person can ingest too much thyroid hormone (overmedication).

Thyroid hormone overproduction

The most common cause of thyroid hormone overproduction is called Graves' disease, another autoimmune endocrine disease. Unlike most other autoimmune diseases (which cause gland hypofunction), Graves' disease results in hyperfunction. An antibody is directed against the TSH receptor in the thyroid cell membrane, stimulating thyroid gland growth and function; this "thyroid-stimulating immunoglobulin (TSIg)" against the receptor mimics TSH (an "imposter" TSH). Although TSH levels are low, the thyroid thinks it is being stimulated (because of the TSH-like properties of the thyroid receptor antibodies).

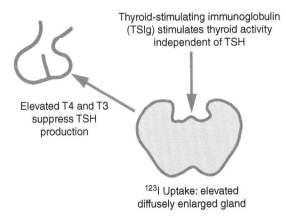

Thyroid-stimulating immunoglobulin (TSIg) stimulates thyroid activity independent of TSH

Elevated T4 and T3 suppress TSH production

^{123}I Uptake: elevated diffusely enlarged gland

Graves' Disease

Thyroid nodules also may "go haywire" and make too much thyroid hormone, resulting in hyperthyroidism. A single nodule may be the culprit (toxic nodule), or multiple nodules may be responsible (toxic multinodular goiter). ("Goiter" is a generic term for thyroid enlargement. The whole thyroid may be enlarged (diffuse goiter), or be nodular (nodular goiter); toxic (hyperthyroid) or nontoxic (euthyroid).) A toxic nodular goiter is like a renegade player who ignores the plays called by the quarterback (the pituitary gland); these tumors seem to have genetic mutations that cause this problem. Even though TSH levels are low, they continue misbehaving as they fail to follow the normal feedback inhibitory mechanisms.

A radioiodine uptake and scan is often performed to verify this type of hyperthyroidism. Those with Graves' disease have a diffusely increased uptake (diffuse toxic goiter), whereas those with hyperfunctioning nodules have scans with a nodular pattern (with suppression of the neighboring normal thyroid tissue, which is "turned off" because of low TSH).

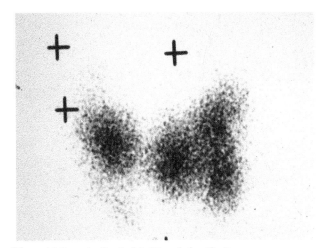

Thyroid Scan in Toxic Multinodular Goiter

The treatment of this type of hyperthyroidism (overproduction) aims to get the thyroid to "slow down." There are three ways to accomplish this. The first is to surgically remove the thyroid. This may be preferred in some instances (i.e., large toxic multinodular goiter causing airway obstruction), but thyroidectomy is not always advised because of the small risk of damaging other delicate structures in the neck. Another way is to give medications that hinder thyroid hormone synthesis. The two antithyroid medications that accomplish this are the thionamide drugs propylthiouracil (PTU) and methimazole. These medications are similar to the compounds (thioureas) found in cabbage and Brussels sprouts (family *Brassicaceae*), and taste bitter to many people. (Historically, the ability to taste the major component of thioureas (phenylthiocarbamide, PTC) produced by the brassicales was one of the earliest demonstrated examples of classical Mendelian inheritance; it is an autosomal dominant trait, and about 70% of people are PTC "tasters.") In fact, these foods contain enough active thiourea compounds to cause thyroid dysfunction if eaten in extremely large amounts (but not in a normal diet).

These drugs generally only work as long as the patient is taking them, although some patients may spontaneously go into remission. Some experts have proposed immune-modifying effects of these drugs.

Most patients tolerate these drugs well. Methimazole is generally preferred to PTU as the former has fewer side effects (except in the first trimester of pregnancy, when PTU is preferred, due to the rare incidence of early birth defects with methimazole; after the first trimester, methimazole is typically used). One potentially life-threatening complication of thionamide treatment is agranulocytosis, when the body ceases to produce the necessary neutrophil cells to fight infection. This occurs in approximately 1 in 500 individuals and can be fatal if the drug is not discontinued; fortunately, most patients recover if the drug is promptly discontinued. Other, less severe side effects (e.g., rash, pruritus) are more common. Liver function test abnormalities are also occasionally seen.

Another type of medication we often give patients with hyperthyroidism is the β-blocker. Remember that one of the effects of thyroid hormone is to stimulate the sympathetic nervous system (resulting in tremors and tachycardia). β-Blockers (e.g., propranolol, metoprolol) decrease the systemic effects of thyroid hormones and alleviate symptoms very quickly. Since they block the adrenergic effects of thyroid hormones and therefore are not dependent on the etiology of the hyperthyroidism, they are useful for all forms of hyperthyroidism. They do not, obviously, treat the cause of hyperthyroidism, they only treat the symptoms; but they are essential adjuncts to therapy, nevertheless.

The third method of treating this type of hyperthyroidism is to employ radioactive iodine (^{131}I). Treatment results in destruction of thyroid tissue and restoration of normal thyroid (euthyroid) hormone levels. Often, the radioactive iodine does *too* much damage, resulting in permanent hypothyroidism. Fortunately, this is easily and inexpensively treated. You might ask, with the vast technical expertise available to us in the 21st century, why we cannot give *just enough* radioactive iodine to render the patient euthyroid. In theory, this would be a good idea—in practice, however, this usually does not work well. If we give too little radioactive iodine, the patient often ends up relapsing (the thyroid has immense potential for growth; even though the patient may have

remained euthyroid for a while after the initial therapy, remaining tissue may again grow, resulting in hyperthyroidism), requiring a second or third treatment. So hypothyroidism is, in most cases, considered almost a desirable result of radioiodine treatment.

Extrathyroidal problems may occur in patients with Graves' disease. The antibodies may stimulate growth of other tissues in addition to the thyroid. The most common associated condition is exophthalmos, which causes protrusion of the eyes (proptosis) and inflammation of the extraocular muscles. This condition may result in impaired eye movement and loss of visual acuity; permanent visual impairment may result in severe cases. Fortunately, most patients with proptosis do not progress to develop significant eye problems. Patients with Graves' disease should always see an eye specialist on a routine basis.

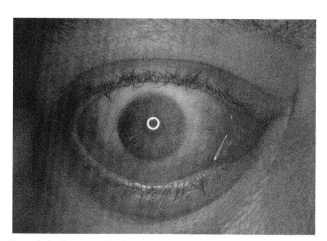

Exophthalmos in Patient with Graves' Disease

Because exophthalmos is caused by thyroid–receptor antibodies with extrathyroidal effects (and not elevated thyroid hormone levels), treatment of the hyperthyroidism does not necessarily improve eye disease. The antibodies are unaffected by treating the thyroid problem with any of the three methods mentioned above (some feel that radioiodine may even make eye disease worse, as therapy results in inflammation and release of massive amounts of antigen into the bloodstream, theoretically worsening the antibody response). Therefore, many experts do not treat patients with severe orbitopathy with radioiodine; pretreatment with corticosteroids may alleviate this potential inflammatory response.

Treatment of exophthalmos includes orbital radiation, extraocular muscle surgery, orbital decompression (to give the eye more room), and corticosteroids (which decrease inflammation). Plasmapheresis (removal of the antibody from serum) can be done in severe cases at specialized medical centers.

A much less common condition occurring in patients with Graves' disease is pretibial myxedema, which results in pebbly orange skin on the shin areas. This is usually a minor problem and does not cause significant disability in most cases. Thyroid acropachy, a disfiguring clubbing of the fingers, may rarely be seen.

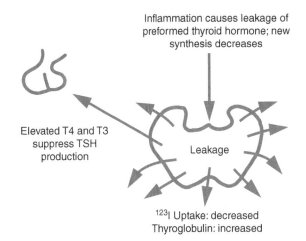

Destructive Thyroiditis

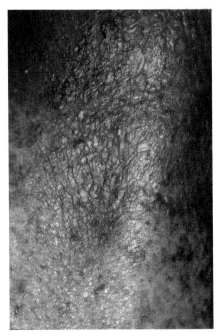

Pretibial Myxedema

Release of preformed thyroid hormone

The thyroid is like a big "water tank" with vast stores of thyroid hormone, contained in the proteinaceous colloid. This is unlike most endocrine glands that do not contain large stores of their hormones. These stores of thyroid hormone are often enough to last for several weeks. Thus, if some mechanism irritates the thyroid so that hormone can "leak out," hyperthyroidism results. This is obviously a different mechanism than thyroid hormone overproduction; it is essential to understand the distinction, as the treatment is different.

One type of thyroid "irritation" (resulting in leakage of preformed hormone) is called subacute thyroiditis. It is often accompanied by pain in the thyroid gland. "Silent thyroiditis" is similar, except that it is without pain. A variant, occurring in about 5% of postpartum women, is called postpartum thyroiditis. The majority of patients with destructive thyroiditis have some type

of underlying autoimmune dysfunction of the thyroid, and some will progress to overt dysfunction in time.

Leakage of stored thyroid hormone results in increased T4 and T3 levels, low TSH, and symptoms of hyperthyroidism. Since new thyroid hormone is not being produced, the uptake of radioiodine is diminished; this is an important way of differentiating destructive thyroiditis from overproduction. This results in the seemingly confusing association of low radioiodine uptake and hyperthyroidism. When you think about the physiology, however, it makes sense (in case you have not noticed, a recurring theme in this text is that the key to mastering endocrinology is to understand physiological pathways rather than memorizing facts). In contrast, in cases of hyperthyroidism due to thyroid hormone overproduction, the thyroid uptake is elevated.

We cannot do a whole lot about thyroid hormone that has already been synthesized; it is there, and we have to deal with it. Antithyroid drugs such as methimazole have no effect, since no new hormone is being made (PTU has a small adjunct effect of decreasing T4 to T3 conversion, but it is not useful enough in this regard to be considered an appropriate therapy for destructive thyroiditis). Radioiodine therapy also would be useless here, since uptake is low and the thyroid would not accumulate a significant amount of ^{131}I; it would merely be excreted. Removing the thyroid surgically is not a good idea either, since this procedure might irritate the thyroid even more and release more stored hormone into the circulation. β-blockers help with the sympathetic symptoms and are used routinely. Nonsteroidal anti-inflammatory agents (e.g., ibuprofen) or corticosteroids decrease inflammation and may be useful in decreasing the leakage.

Fortunately, like a water tank that springs a leak, there is only a finite amount of substance inside, which will eventually run out. Thyroid hormone levels in time will actually drop below normal, producing a temporary state of hypothyroidism. It may take several weeks for the thyroid to rebuild its stores, at which time the patient again becomes euthyroid (leading to the typical triphasic "hyperthyroid–hypothyroid–euthyroid" course of this disorder). Rarely, in destructive thyroiditis, the inflammation is so severe that the thyroid cannot regenerate completely, resulting in permanent hypothyroidism. This is easily treated with daily thyroxine replacement.

Exogenous ingestion of thyroid hormone
Another cause of thyrotoxicosis with low radioiodine uptake occurs in those who take too much thyroid hormone because the dosage of thyroxine is too high. It can also occur in people who illicitly take thyroid hormone, often in an effort to lose weight. This most commonly occurs in health care providers with access to readily available thyroid hormone.

Another interesting example of this type of thyrotoxicosis occurred many years ago. Remember that an early therapy for hypothyroidism was the ingestion of animal thyroid glands. It appears that, in one part of the country, a batch of hamburger was made from beef in which the thyroid glands had not been removed. The thyroid glands were ground up with hamburger resulting in large amounts of T4, which survived cooking and resulted in thyrotoxicosis in many patients. This phenomenon was appropriately termed "hamburger thyrotoxicosis."

It is important to distinguish this type of thyrotoxicosis from the type already discussed that presents with a low radioiodine uptake (destructive thyroiditis). Remember how thyroxine is stored in the colloid, attached to a protein called thyroglobulin (Tg). (Do not be confused between the protein Tg (thyroglobulin) and the carrier protein thyroid-binding globulin (TBG).) With thyroiditis and release of thyroid hormone, the thyroglobulin is released into the bloodstream too, resulting in an increased Tg level. Those who take too much hormone have low Tg levels, since Tg is not contained in the thyroxine tablet. While we should hope that patients would be forthcoming regarding ingestion of exogenous T4, such is not always the case.

Secondary hyperthyroidism
As we discussed above, secondary hyperthyroidism is quite rare. TSH-secreting pituitary tumors produce elevated TSH and T4 levels. This condition is readily distinguished from primary hyperthyroidism by the inappropriately elevated TSH levels in the presence of elevated peripheral levels (in Graves' disease and other causes of primary hyperthyroidism, TSH should be low). Treatment includes medication (octreotide) and/or surgical resection. Antithyroid drugs and/or radioiodine do not treat the cause and may actually make the problem (the pituitary tumor) worse.

Another, very rare cause of secondary hyperthyroidism is pituitary thyroid hormone resistance, an inherited disorder in which the pituitary is resistant to levels of T4 and T3 in the circulation. Since TSH does not suppress normally, it continues stimulating the thyroid and hyperthyroidism may result.

Severe thyrotoxicosis: thyroid storm
Thyroid storm is a condition caused by severe thyrotoxicosis. Graves' disease is the typical cause, and other forms of hyperthyroidism only rarely result in symptoms of this degree. These persons present with fever, confusion, and severe tachycardia, and may suffer cardiovascular collapse. The mortality rate is high if untreated. Treatment includes β-blockers and antithyroid drugs.

THYROID NODULES

A goiter is a generic term for any thyroid enlargement. Goiters may be diffuse as in Graves' disease, or nodular. Nodular goiters are common, especially in women. A patient may have either a single (solitary) nodule or multiple nodules (multinodular goiter). They are usually euthyroid, although hypo- or hyperthyroidism may also be associated with thyroid nodules, as we have discussed. The main concern is whether the nodule is benign or malignant.

Fortunately, most thyroid nodules are benign, especially those that have remained unchanged for years. Those that are rapidly growing are more likely to be malignant. In the glorious "atomic age" of the 1950s, doctors gave radiation treatments for a variety of benign conditions ranging from acne to enlarged tonsils. We know now that these seemingly innocuous "radiation treatments" caused more problems than they cured, and resulted in a small increase in the incidence of thyroid cancer (as well as an increased incidence of cancer in those physicians who used such devices without adequate shielding); therefore, a careful history must be obtained from each patient.

How do we efficiently evaluate thyroid nodules, since they are so common? We do not want to miss a malignancy, but we also do not want to expose patients to potentially painful and pricey procedures, unless clearly necessary. A costly evaluation method is to perform a radionuclide thyroid scan. A nodule may not concentrate radioiodine as well as the surrounding thyroid tissue, leading to a "punched out" or "cold" nodule appearance on the scan. If it concentrates radioiodine as well, it cannot be distinguished from normal thyroid and is called "warm." A hyperfunctioning nodule ("hot nodule") suppresses the surrounding thyroid tissue.

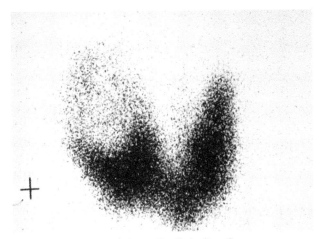

"Cold" Thyroid Nodule on Radioiodine Scan

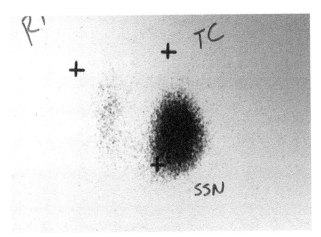

Hyperfunctioning or "Hot" Thyroid Nodule on Radioiodine Scan

Unfortunately, this information is really not very useful to us. It is a common belief that "cold nodules" are usually malignant, but this is not true. They are somewhat more likely to be malignant than hot nodules, but most cold nodules (at least 80%) are benign. Some also erroneously think that hot nodules can never be cancerous, but carcinoma can (very rarely) arise in such nodules. So, as a result, it turns out that a nuclear thyroid scan is just not very useful in evaluating euthyroid or hypothyroid patients with thyroid nodules.

A better way of delineating anatomy is to perform a thyroid ultrasound. This can demonstrate the depth of a nodule (whereas a radionuclide scan only yields a poor quality, two-dimensional frontal picture). Pure cystic (fluid-filled) and "spongiform" nodules are less likely to be malignant than solid ones. Mixed cystic-solid nodules, hypoechoic nodules (those that appear "dark" on ultrasound), and those with microcalcifications are more likely to be malignant.

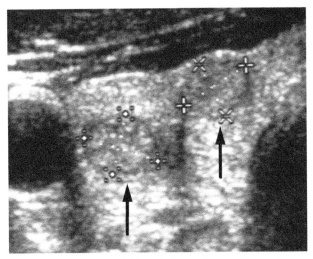

Ultrasound of Thyroid Nodule in Patient with Papillary Thyroid Carcinoma

So, to truly know the nature and size of the nodules, an ultrasound is the way to go, and it does give us more information than the nuclear scan—but still does not definitively answer what we need to know.

Well, we have not yet mentioned a really good way to distinguish benign from malignant nodules, and we really need a better test. The best way today is to actually look at thyroid cells under a microscope, by a procedure called fine needle aspiration (FNA). The advent of genetic testing for markers predisposing for thyroid cancer (BRAF, PAX/PPAR-γ, etc.) has much promise in helping identifying patients at high risk (and excluding those at low risk from unnecessary surgery), thus creating a more scientifically advanced approach to management. But a biopsy must still be done in many circumstances; this is done with a very small needle as an outpatient, and causes minimal discomfort to the patient. Ultrasound may be used to guide the needle with nodules that are difficult to feel. The sensitivity (ability of the test to detect cancer in those with the disease) is about 95–98% in the hands of a skilled clinician and cytopathologist. Genetic markers are of greatest use in identifying high-risk patients with "indeterminate" results on fine needle biopsy, where malignancy cannot be completely excluded.

If the nodule is malignant, it should obviously be removed. If it is benign, no treatment is necessary (although it may need to be removed if it causes hoarseness, cosmetic disfigurement, etc.). Unfortunately, many biopsies fall somewhere in the middle with "nondiagnostic" or "suspicious" features that neither confirm nor refute the diagnosis of malignancy. Some seemingly benign tumors (e.g., follicular adenomas) should be removed, because they may harbor occult cancerous cells. Suppression with thyroxine has been employed in the past, but recent studies show that this treatment is of no benefit and may even be harmful. Benign nodules that are cosmetically disfiguring may be removed. Others are simply followed with regular examinations.

DIFFERENTIATED (EPITHELIAL) THYROID CARCINOMA

The words "carcinoma" and "cancer" sound ominous to any patient or clinician, for obvious reasons. Fortunately, the most common types of thyroid cancer grow very slowly and rarely cause death. These are the epithelial thyroid cancers (papillary and follicular cancer) and account for 95% of those with thyroid cancer. They are called epithelial thyroid cancers because they arise from follicular epithelium and not from other cells within the thyroid. Papillary is the most common type of thyroid carcinoma. No one obviously wants to have cancer, but if you had to pick a malignancy to have, this is probably the type to get. Most patients have lesions confined to the thyroid. Rarely, metastases and death occur, usually many years after diagnosis and treatment. Follicular cancer is a bit more aggressive than papillary, but most patients do well and often survive for many years even with distant metastases.

The cornerstone of treatment of epithelial thyroid cancers is removal of the thyroid. The majority of patients are cured by this treatment alone. After the thyroid has been completely removed by the surgeon, all the cancer is usually gone. The method by which we follow this type of cancer, however, necessitates another type of treatment. We follow thyroid cancer by two means: (a) radioiodine scanning or (b) serum thyroglobulin (Tg) levels. The scan will not work properly, however, until every last bit of the thyroid is gone. If there is even a microscopic amount of normal thyroid left (called "remnants"), it will take up the tracer rather than the possible tumor, and the scan will be fruitless. We measure Tg, since it is a marker of thyroid epithelial tissue—if levels go up it means the cancer could be coming back. However, the thyroid remnant makes Tg too, and we cannot distinguish Tg of normal thyroid epithelial origin from that of cancer tissue origin.

Therefore, we must get rid of these small remnants in order to see a tumor in the patient's body or rely on serum Tg levels. This is easily done with a high-dose ^{131}I treatment, which basically burns up the small remaining pieces. Only after these are gone can we later do a reliable scan to look for metastases (which hopefully are not there). This therapy is called a "remnant ablation." This is the same type of radioiodine used for hyperthyroidism, but is given in a higher dose.

The treatment itself is very simple. It involves swallowing a radioactive iodine capsule, similar to the thyroid scan. It is painless and does not involve intravenous lines or injections. Radioactive iodine usually does not cause side effects, and the radiation dose to the rest of the patient's body is quite small. Patients do not experience hair loss, nausea, or vomiting that can occur with other types of cancer therapy. Occasionally there is some tenderness in the neck area (radiation thyroiditis). They also might experience an unusual taste in their mouths or swelling of the salivary glands, which usually only lasts a few days.

While we used to treat all thyroid cancer patients with remnant ablation, we no longer do this for patients deemed "low risk" (i.e., small tumor size, no lymph node involvement or extension through the capsule, etc.). We also use lower doses (e.g., 30 mCi) than in years past (100–150 mCi was the common "standard"). So it is no longer the "standard of care" it once was for many patients.

Some patients need follow-up with whole-body nuclear scans (^{123}I). Before the thyroid cancer survey, all thyroid hormone has to be out of the patient's system. This is because thyroid cancer cells are relatively insensitive

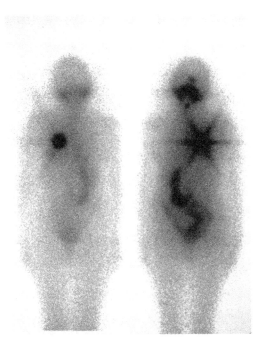

Pulmonary Metastasis on Radioiodine Scan in Patients with Follicular Thyroid Carcinoma

to radioiodine, and high TSH levels must be present to stimulate cancer cells, if present, to take up the isotope. Can you think of a simple way to cause elevated TSH levels in a patient without a thyroid? The obvious method is to induce hypothyroidism by taking the patient off his or her thyroid hormone. The patient must discontinue thyroxine for several weeks for this to occur. Regrettably, this causes patients to develop significant symptoms of hypothyroidism and feel very poorly (this may even be a health hazard in patients with other debilitating conditions).

Since the only reason to discontinue the thyroid hormone is to achieve high TSH levels, you might ask why we cannot just give TSH to the patients to alleviate their discomfort. In the past, this was impossible because TSH was not available. Today, however, synthetic human TSH (of recombinant DNA origin) is readily available (albeit expensive), and can be given to patients via an injection before the scan, eliminating the need to stop thyroid hormone in many patients.

A follow-up scan may be done in a year or two. Serum thyroglobulin (Tg) levels are also monitored, and hopefully will be low (indicating negligible thyroid epithelial cell mass).

If a scan shows metastases or Tg levels rise, a repeat high-dose radioiodine therapy may be necessary. For patients with advanced disease, drugs such as sunitinib (a tyrosine kinase inhibitor) may be useful.

MEDULLARY AND ANAPLASTIC THYROID CARCINOMA

Medullary thyroid carcinoma (MTC) is a less common type of thyroid cancer arising in the parafollicular (C) cells of the thyroid, which manufacture the hormone calcitonin. This is a much more aggressive form of thyroid cancer, and those with widespread metastases have a poor prognosis. This type of tumor does not make thyroglobulin and does not concentrate radioiodine well, so treatment with the latter is usually ineffective. Serum calcitonin levels are usually elevated, and useful to follow as a marker of tumor burden. Treatment with external radiation therapy and/or chemotherapy may offer palliative benefit in those with severe disease.

Anaplastic carcinoma is by far the most aggressive thyroid cancer, and one of the most lethal of all cancers. It presents as rapid thyroid enlargement, often over a matter of days. There is no universally effective treatment (although many clinical trials are underway), and most patients die within weeks to months. This type of tumor is not responsive to radioactive iodine.

REVIEW QUESTIONS

1. A 32-year-old woman presents with a 3-month history of irregular menses, dry skin, and mild hair loss. She has a small goiter on examination, and her weight is up 12 lb from her last visit with you a year ago (BMI is now 24 mg/kg^2). Serum TSH is moderately elevated at 22.3 mIU/mL (N: 0.3–5.0 mIU/mL). Skin is moderately dry, and her vital signs are normal.

   a. What is the probable diagnosis?
   b. Are there any additional tests you would want to order?
   c. What would be the treatment?
   d. How soon would you see her back to re-check levels and monitor progress?

(a) This is a classic presentation of primary hypothyroidism. The elevated TSH is consistent with this.

(b) While measuring peripheral hormone levels (free T4) and antithyroid peroxidase (TPO) antibodies could be done, they likely will be abnormal and would add little to the diagnosis.

(c) The treatment of choice would be synthetic levothyroxine at a dose appropriate for her body size.

(d) Thyroxine has a half-life of approximately 1 week, so it would take at least four half-lives (1 month) to reach a steady-state concentration. Therefore, seeing her back in 6 weeks is reasonable. A common error is seeing the patient back too soon (e.g., 2 weeks) and increasing the dosage because the levels have not normalized.

2. A 37-year-old female presents with a "swelling" in her left anterior neck. Upon palpation, you discover a 2.5 × 3 cm freely movable thyroid nodule near the midline. Thyroid functions (TSH and T4) are normal. Ultrasound demonstrates the palpable nodule with no other nodules noted; the nodule is cystic in consistency. The next best strategy in management of this nodule is:
   a. Surgical removal (left hemithyroidectomy)
   b. Radionuclide (^{123}I) thyroid scan
   c. Fine needle aspiration (FNA)
   d. Observation and repeat ultrasound in 1 year

(c) This is a fairly large nodule and malignancy should be excluded. While the ultrasound characteristics (cystic) favor benign pathology and observation (d), FNA is likely warranted. (Smaller nodules might be simply observed.) She should not undergo a major surgical procedure (a) without further evidence of malignancy. Radioiodine scans (b) are of minimal use in evaluating euthyroid nodules.

3. A 33-year-old woman presents with a 6-week history of 20 lb (9 kg) weight loss, nervousness, palpitations, and heat intolerance. She takes no medications other than an oral contraceptive. Examination reveals a thin woman with extremely soft skin, large diffuse goiter (three times normal size), and mild proptosis. What is the likely diagnosis?
   a. Hashimoto's thyroiditis

   b. Toxic multinodular goiter
   c. Surreptitious ingestion of exogenous thyroid hormone
   d. Graves' disease
   e. There is insufficient information to make the diagnosis

(d) This is a classic presentation of diffuse toxic goiter (Graves' disease); she has typical symptoms of thyrotoxicosis with proptosis (seen only in Graves' disease) and diffuse goiter. The excessively soft skin is due to high epidermal turnover; in contrast, patients with hypothyroidism often have dry skin due to low turnover. Hashimoto's thyroiditis (a) usually presents with hypothyroidism, but can present on occasion with a transient thyrotoxic phase (a form of destructive thyroiditis), but without proptosis. There are no nodules palpated on examination (b). Patients with factitious thyrotoxicosis (c) would not have a goiter, as TSH suppression would cause thyroid atrophy.

4. A 23-year-old woman who just gave birth to her first infant 2 months ago presents with mild tachycardia and a 10-lb (4.5 kg) weight loss. She takes no medications. She does not have proptosis or a goiter. Serum free T4 is elevated, and serum TSH is suppressed. A 24-h uptake of ^{123}I is suppressed at 3% (normal: 20–35%). She is breastfeeding the infant and does not want to take any medications unless absolutely necessary. The best treatment for her disorder is:
   a. Methimazole
   b. Observation
   c. Radioiodine (^{131}I)
   d. Toxic nodular goiter

(b) This is a classic presentation of postpartum thyroiditis, a form of destructive thyroiditis occurring in approximately 5% of postpartum women. As with most cases of destructive thyroiditis, it is a self-limited disorder. Methimazole (a) and radioiodine (c) are not appropriate treatments for destructive thyroiditis; ^{131}I is also absolutely contraindicated in breastfeeding women. β-Blockers might be considered to help symptoms (and are generally safe in breastfeeding), but she does not desire medication.

Adrenal Gland

In the previous lecture we learned about our first major endocrine system controlled by the hypothalamus and pituitary—the thyroid gland. This gland is of paramount importance because of the thyroid's diverse effects on other organ systems.

T4 (tetraiodothyronine) is the major thyroid hormone secreted by the thyroid. It is made up of two modified tyrosine molecules with four iodine atoms attached. T3 (triiodothyronine) is the most potent thyroid hormone and is primarily made by the peripheral conversion of T4 in the peripheral circulation by a deiodinase (although the thyroid does secrete a small amount of T3). The trophic hormone for T4 production is the pituitary hormone TSH. Under the influence of TSH, iodine is trapped (actively transported into the epithelial cell), organified (attached to the thyronine molecules), and stored within the functional unit of the thyroid (follicle) in colloid, attached to a protein called thyroglobulin. When needed, T4 is secreted from the colloid into the bloodstream.

Common measurements of thyroid function include the iodothyronines T4 and T3, as well as pituitary TSH. The thyroid scan is a common nuclear medicine study. This is an image of the thyroid taken after administration of radioactive iodine. A thyroid uptake is the fractional accumulation of radioactive iodine after a set period of time, accounting for the amount lost by natural decay. ^{123}I is most commonly used for imaging; ^{131}I is used for destroying thyroid tissue (e.g., hyperthyroidism and thyroid cancer).

Hypothyroidism is one of the most common endocrine diseases. The most common cause is the autoimmune disorder Hashimoto's thyroiditis. In primary hypothyroidism, TSH levels rise in an effort to stimulate the thyroid. The elevated TSH level, therefore, is the most sensitive indicator of hypothyroidism. Symptoms of hypothyroidism include cold intolerance, dry skin, muscle cramps, slowed mentation, irregular menses in women, and constipation. Untreated hypothyroidism in children results in a serious condition called cretinism. Fortunately, hypothyroidism is inexpensively and easily treated with thyroid hormone. Synthetic thyroxine is the treatment of choice.

Thyrotoxicosis is the condition of thyroid hormone excess and has a variety of causes (endogenous and exogenous). Hyperthyroidism is a subset of thyrotoxicosis that originates from the patient's thyroid (endogenous). The first type results from production of too much thyroid hormone. The most common cause is Graves' disease, which also is an autoimmune disease. It is unique in that it is one of the few autoimmune diseases that results in endocrine excess (most cause deficiency). Thyroid nodules that produce too much thyroid hormone (toxic adenoma or toxic multinodular goiter) are another common cause of thyroid hormone overproduction. These tumors usually have germline mutations that render them unresponsive to regulation by TSH. Treatment of this type of hyperthyroidism includes antithyroid medication, radioactive iodine therapy, or surgery.

Hyperthyroidism may also be caused by leakage of preformed thyroid hormone. This is illustrated by destructive thyroiditis, in which irritation of the thyroid leads to spillage of preformed hormone. In contrast to thyroid hormone overproduction, the thyroid uptake in this type of hyperthyroidism is decreased. This type of hyperthyroidism normally resolves on its own. Another cause of thyrotoxicosis is the ingestion of too much thyroid hormone. This usually occurs in individuals who are trying to lose weight or have psychiatric problems (factitious) or in persons inadvertently prescribed too much medication by their provider (iatrogenic).

Thyroid nodules are quite common, especially in women. Most often they are benign. Radionuclide thyroid scans are generally a poor modality for evaluating thyroid nodules, since they do not reliably distinguish benign from malignant lesions and provide limited two-dimensional anatomic information. Ultrasound is a far better way to discern anatomy, and some ultrasonic criteria help the clinician distinguish benign from malignant lesions. The best way, however, to distinguish a benign from a malignant thyroid nodule is to perform a fine needle aspiration biopsy. Genetic markers of thyroid cancer are being used as another way to classify "indeterminate" neoplasms that may be at high risk for malignancy, to help low-risk patients avoid unnecessary surgery.

Thyroid carcinomas may be divided into two types: carcinomas arising from epithelial tissue (papillary and follicular carcinoma) and the non-epithelial varieties (medullary and anaplastic carcinoma); these definitions exclude metastatic cancer from other sites. Epithelial thyroid carcinomas are treated by surgical excision and radioactive iodine therapy. The other types of thyroid cancer do not respond to radioactive iodine, and surgery is the mainstay of therapy; treatment of these (especially anaplastic) is often palliative.

THE ADRENAL GLANDS

In this lecture we will study the adrenal glands, which are often called the "fight or flight" glands because they secrete hormones necessary for homeostasis under physical stress. In our football team analogy, they are like the running back or wide receiver who is capable of blocking (i.e., support services to other players), but also capable of accelerating many times normal speed to break the big play when needed. The adrenals are paired glands that lie in the retroperitoneal cavity above the kidneys. They have two functional parts—most of the adrenal consists of the outer cortex, with the remainder being the inner medulla.

The adrenal cortex contains three layers, or zones, and makes steroid hormones, which are derived from cholesterol. The only other organs that synthesize steroids are the gonads (ovaries and testes), which make sex steroids. The outermost cortical layer, called the zona glomerulosa, is responsible for synthesizing steroids that help us retain salt and water; hence this layer's principal steroid, aldosterone, is called a mineralocorticoid. This hormone is necessary for life.

The thickest or middle layer, the zona fasciculata, makes another life-sustaining group of hormones, the glucocorticoids. As the name implies, these compounds are important in helping the body maintain adequate glucose (energy) levels. The major glucocorticoid of interest is cortisol (hydrocortisone).

The thinnest cortical layer is the innermost (the zona fasciculata), which provides adrenal androgen secretion in both men and women. Most testosterone in the male originates from the testes, however. These hormones are not necessary to sustain life.

The inner medulla is the site of catecholamine synthesis. The catecholamine hormones (e.g., epinephrine) are important during stressful physiologic situations.

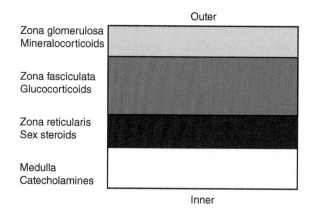

Adrenal Cortex and Medulla

All steroids are synthesized from cholesterol. For cholesterol to be useful, it must be transported to the mitochondria by steroidogenic acute regulatory protein (StAR). In the mitochondrion, cholesterol is converted to pregnenolone by the cholesterol side-chain cleavage enzyme. All steroids of the cortex are made from pregnenolone by a variety of different enzymes (see the following figure). Most of these are in the family of cytochrome P450 oxygenases. Drugs that inhibit enzymes in the P450 system (e.g., ketoconazole, etomidate) may inhibit steroid synthesis.

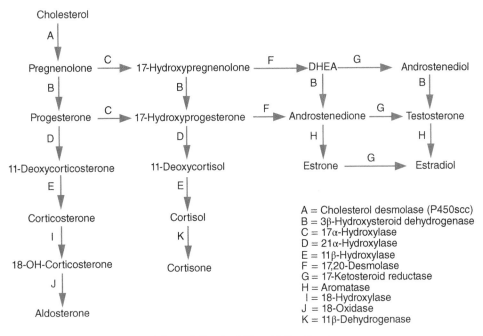

Adrenal Cortical Steroid Synthesis

A = Cholesterol desmolase (P450scc)
B = 3β-Hydroxysteroid dehydrogenase
C = 17α-Hydroxylase
D = 21α-Hydroxylase
E = 11β-Hydroxylase
F = 17,20-Desmolase
G = 17-Ketosteroid reductase
H = Aromatase
 I = 18-Hydroxylase
J = 18-Oxidase
K = 11β-Dehydrogenase

Let us discuss the glucocorticoids first. Although all adrenal steroids are made in the cortex, glucocorticoids are sometimes called corticosteroids because of their necessity for life (and the fact that the zona fasciculata is the thickest layer). Their name is derived from their ability to increase glucose concentrations via increased gluconeogenesis and decreased glucose uptake. They are therefore activated when the body is in a fasting state or otherwise needs energy. Life is not possible without normal amounts of these hormones. In excess amounts, however, they inhibit protein synthesis and promote protein breakdown, since they are meant to help the body obtain energy. The primary glucocorticoid of interest is cortisol (hydrocortisone).

Like most endocrine organs, the zona fasciculata is under control by a feedback loop. It and the zona reticularis—site of male hormone (androgen) synthesis—are essentially separate organs from the aldosterone-synthesizing glomerulosa, and are under different control. The stimulus for the zona fasciculata is the anterior pituitary hormone ACTH (adrenocorticotropic hormone, corticotropin). Under stimulation

Major Adrenal Cortical Steroids

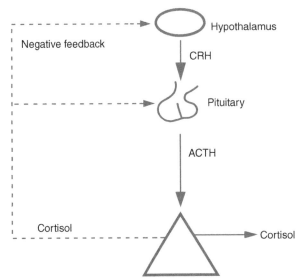

Normal Adrenal Axis

by ACTH, this layer increases production of its hormone. Minutes after ACTH levels increase, cortisol levels increase; this phenomenon can be observed by measuring serum cortisol levels before and after ACTH infusion.

After cortisol levels reach a certain plateau, this tells the pituitary that there is enough to slow down ACTH production. Under times of stress (e.g., surgery, sepsis, or even strenuous exercise), ACTH levels increase to produce more cortisol (to provide the body with more energy). The body can produce as much as 10 times the normal amount of cortisol, if necessary (approximately 300 mg/day). One of the biggest physiological stresses of all in humans is pregnancy, where cortisol levels can rise to several times the normal.

Cortisol excess: Cushing's syndrome

Normally, this all works quite well, and cortisol levels remain appropriate. But occasionally something goes awry and too much cortisol is produced. This deleterious phenomenon is called Cushing's syndrome (CS) (named after Harvey Cushing, a famous endocrine neurosurgeon), and may have several different causes.

Let us think of the ways that the body could produce too much cortisol. If there is too much ACTH, the cortex would make too much. Cushing's disease is a subtype of Cushing's syndrome caused by an ACTH-secreting pituitary tumor. This is the most common cause (about 2/3 of cases) of endogenous CS (i.e., the source of cortisol originates within the body).

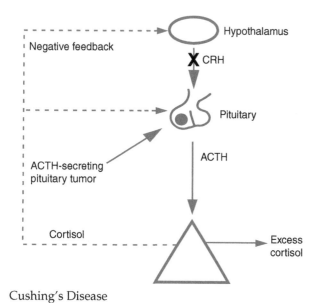

Cushing's Disease

There are other tumors that can also make ACTH. These include neuroendocrine tumors such as small

cell lung carcinoma, which can manufacture other neuroendocrine peptides (e.g., antidiuretic hormone). Pheochromocytomas can rarely make ACTH. Since here the source of ACTH is outside its native source (the pituitary), this syndrome is called "ectopic" (paraneoplastic or "out of place") ACTH syndrome. (More on this later.) This is the second most common cause of endogenous CS. In these causes of CS, the ACTH level is elevated, often hundreds to thousands of times normal in ectopic ACTH syndrome, which tends to be much more aggressive than Cushing's disease. Indeed, because of the aggressive nature of these malignancies, a presenting sign of ectopic ACTH syndrome may be cachexia and electrolyte abnormalities rather than the typical morphological findings often associated with CS (discussed shortly).

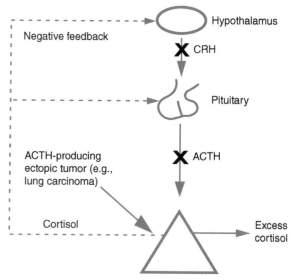

Ectopic ACTH Syndrome

CS may also occur if the adrenal goes "haywire" and makes too much cortisol on its own, without regulation by ACTH. This type occurs with tumors that do not respond to normal feedback (again, a common theme in this book is that all disorders are fundamentally due to disruption of the normal feedback mechanisms discussed in the first chapter). These may be benign tumors (adenomas, more common), or malignant (adrenocortical carcinomas). The latter are rare causes of CS, but tend to be very aggressive and are often fatal. Since the pituitary works normally, ACTH levels are "shut off" (low); this is how these causes can be distinguished from ACTH-dependent causes.

Thus far we have discussed endogenous causes, but, in fact, the most common cause of CS is exogenous (i.e., the source of the steroid is outside the body). Synthetic glucocorticoids are used for many conditions, including chronic rheumatologic and pulmonary disease, and given to those receiving immunosuppression for organ transplants (this is much less common today given improved immunosuppressive regimens, reducing the need for steroids). These persons must receive very high doses of steroids to suppress their disease.

Exogenous CS is usually obvious, since it is usually known to the health care provider that the person is on steroids. Since the pituitary sees too much cortisol, ACTH levels are low (remember the feedback inhibition pathway).

The clinical features of CS are due to the deleterious effects of cortisol excess. Skin strength is diminished, and easy bruising and pigmented striae (stretch marks) are common. Cortisol excess destroys muscle mass, so these people tend to be very weak, especially in the proximal limb muscles. It is common for even a young person with CS to be unable to perform a deep knee bend without assistance. Osteoporosis is common (as excess glucocorticoid decreases bone formation), and a presenting complaint may be a pathologic fracture. They may develop central obesity and a characteristic fat deposition in the cervical area ("buffalo hump"). A round "moon face" is common, although some patients with CS have only mild obesity and do not look like the "classic" patients found in textbooks. As with any clinical encounter establishing a disease's temporal progression, examination of old photographs is crucial, as neither patients nor family members necessarily recall such details accurately, given that the changes can take years to occur.

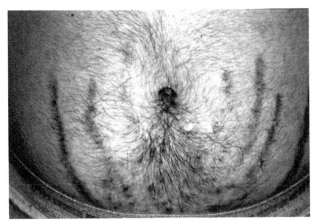

Striae in Patient with Cushing's Syndrome

There are several ways to screen a patient for CS. Because of the periodic nature of ACTH and hence cortisol secretion, random values are often of little value. A tried-and-true screening test is the measurement of urine cortisol excretion over a 24-h period. A normal value rules against CS, while an elevated level warrants further investigation. Another screening test is the dexamethasone suppression test. This test exploits the ability of an administered synthetic glucocorticoid (dexamethasone) to suppress ACTH and cortisol secretion in the normal individual. If we give dexamethasone (1 mg) to a normal person in the evening, the cortisol level should drop very low by the next morning, because of physiologic suppression of ACTH production (1 mg of dexamethasone equals about 30 mg of hydrocortisone in terms of potency, equal to or greater than the average amount secreted per day). Conversely, in the person with CS, the level does not drop. Either the ACTH level does not fall low enough (in the ACTH-dependent forms, Cushing's disease and ectopic ACTH), or the rampant adrenal continues to work on its own (adrenal tumors). This is just a screening test, and like the 24-h urine cortisol test, a confirmatory test is needed.

Another useful screening test is the measurement of salivary cortisol levels. Here, the patient places small cotton plugs in the mouth, and cortisol levels are measured in the evening. This test has shown much promise and may replace some of the cumbersome dexamethasone suppression tests, which sometimes yield confusing results (due to patients not taking the dexamethasone properly), failure to collect urine accurately, presence of drugs that accelerate the metabolism of dexamethasone, making it ineffective (e.g., topiramate), and so on.

The confirmatory test for CS is another type of DST, the low-dose test. In this test, a higher dose of dexamethasone (0.5 mg) is given every 6 h for 2 days, and serum cortisol and urine cortisol levels are measured. In normal persons, the levels suppress; in those with CS, they do not.

Once CS is confirmed, how do we isolate the cause? The ACTH level is valuable here. If elevated, the CS cannot be caused by adrenal tumors, since the high cortisol levels with adrenal CS tell the hypothalamic–pituitary axis (HPA) to shut off. If ACTH is elevated, we are then left with CD versus ectopic ACTH. A pituitary MRI may show a tumor, which suggests CD. A large lung tumor suggests ectopic ACTH syndrome. In cases where these studies are equivocal, a technique called petrosal sinus sampling is done. Here, ACTH is actually measured from the petrosal sinuses (which drain the pituitary) and compared to ACTH in the peripheral blood. Pituitary ACTH levels higher than peripheral levels (greater than twofold) suggest CD. (The gradient is often much higher.) If not, ectopic ACTH syndrome is suggested. If the ACTH level is low, adrenal computed tomography (CT) or MRI may isolate the tumor. Incidentally discovered pituitary tumors are fairly common, and the mere presence of a tumor does not prove it is functioning; therefore, a dynamic assessment of function such as petrosal sinus sampling is often useful and can prevent an unnecessary surgery.

The cause of CS is then treated. For Cushing's disease, the pituitary tumor is removed. With small tumors, this probably will leave normal residual pituitary function. With large tumors, the pituitary may be damaged, requiring hormone replacement. The somatostatin analog pasireotide is an effective treatment for patients with Cushing's disease who have failed surgery or who are poor surgical candidates. The dopamine agonist cabergoline (typically used for prolactinomas) also has a modest effect in those with CD. Therefore, most patients with CD have favorable outcomes.

Unfortunately, ectopic ACTH syndrome is usually not curable because of the aggressive nature of many tumors (small cell lung carcinoma). Some tumors (e.g., bronchial carcinoids) are more indolent. The tumor (e.g., lung cancer) is treated by whatever means necessary, and may be palliative. Drugs that diminish adrenal steroid synthesis (e.g., ketoconazole, mitotane) may be considered.

A novel therapy for patients with CS who have failed conventional treatments is mifepristone (RU-486), a progesterone receptor antagonist originally developed as an abortifacient (as an emergency contraceptive); it also has glucocorticoid receptor antagonist activity at higher concentrations. Mifepristone binds to the glucocorticoid receptor with high affinity, but it has little affinity for the mineralocorticoid receptor. While it does not treat the cause (just like pegvisomant does not treat the GH excess in acromegaly), it blocks the effect of excess glucocorticoids—although the mineralocorticoid effects still may persist.

Adrenal tumors should be surgically removed, since the body can function quite well with only one adrenal gland. Adrenocortical cancers are much more aggressive and may not be curable. Metastases are frequent and often fatal, and drugs such as mitotane may be used as adjuvant therapy. Reducing the dosage of administered glucocorticoid to the lowest possible level can minimize iatrogenic CS.

Adrenocortical insufficiency: Addison's disease

Each endocrine organ has a deficiency syndrome as well as a hormonal excess syndrome. Since the adrenal cortex is necessary for life, it would stand to reason that adrenal insufficiency (AI) would cause many problems. Like all deficiency syndromes, AI may be primary or secondary. Primary AI occurs when the adrenal gland itself is damaged; secondary AI occurs if the cortex has atrophied because of insufficient ACTH.

Primary AI is also called Addison's disease, named after Thomas Addison, who first described the condition in 1849. Like most endocrine deficiency syndromes, the most common cause is autoimmune. Other causes include tuberculosis, congenital adrenal enzyme defects, fungal infection (typically histoplasmosis), infiltrative diseases (hemochromatosis), HIV infection, and metastatic cancer (uncommon; while the adrenals are a frequent site of metastasis, this only rarely causes adrenal insufficiency).

Since cortisol is a stress hormone, it stands to reason that those with AI do not have a lot of energy. Indeed, these persons are frequently weak, anorexic, hypoglycemic, and depressed. As a young man, President John F. Kennedy developed weakness, weight loss, and hyperpigmentation, and he finally was diagnosed as having Addison's disease in 1947. Fortunately for him, cortisone was discovered in 1949 (100 years after Addison described the condition).

In primary endocrine deficiency disorders, the trophic hormone always rises in a futile effort to get the gland working. In this case, ACTH rises, often to hundreds of times above normal. An interesting property of ACTH is its similarity to the hormone melanocyte-stimulating hormone (α-MSH), which is not very important in humans. This hormone is important in many lower vertebrates (e.g., reptiles and amphibians) that change color to blend with their environment and escape predators. In humans, melanocytes are responsible for moles, freckles, and suntan. The very high ACTH levels in Addison's disease act like MSH and cause increased melanin deposition and hyperpigmentation in the skin. (MSH, however, has no ACTH-like activity.) Indeed, those with Addison's disease often look like they just came in from weeks in the Florida sun. In fact, early on in the disease, some patients are actually pleased because they lose weight and have a nice suntan, without any effort (or the risks associated with excessive sun exposure)! This is not a good way to get a tan, though, as patients eventually become ill and seek medical treatment; death can occur in cases of concurrent catastrophic illness.

You might ask if those with Cushing's disease or ectopic ACTH syndrome develop hyperpigmentation. Those with Cushing's disease usually do not have sufficiently high ACTH levels to develop this problem, but levels may be high enough in ectopic ACTH syndrome to cause it.

There are many common laboratory abnormalities in those with Addison's disease. Since cortisol is important for glucose metabolism, hypoglycemia may be seen. Aldosterone is important in helping the body get rid of potassium and hold onto sodium, and hyperkalemia and hyponatremia are often seen. Cortisol is also important in helping the body hold onto sodium. Patients may be dehydrated, so serum blood urea nitrogen (BUN) and creatinine may be elevated.

Patients may go on for years with mild disease and only minor symptoms. Often, it is suspected because the person fails to recover from minor illnesses easily (e.g., viral infections) or becomes ill during stress (e.g., pregnancy). If subjected to enough stress, adrenal crisis or shock may result. This can happen if the previously undiagnosed AI sufferer is in an accident, undergoes surgery, or has a serious illness (e.g., myocardial infarction), which precipitates the adrenal crisis.

Fortunately, Addison's disease (primary adrenal insufficiency) is easily and inexpensively treated. Cortisone was isolated in 1949 and was deemed a "wonder drug," although we know now that too much of it is harmful. Patients with Addison's disease receive an oral glucocorticoid, such as the naturally occurring hydrocortisone or cortisone. (Cortisone is itself biologically inert, and must undergo hepatic conversion to hydrocortisone.) Alternatively, a synthetic glucocorticoid such as prednisone or dexamethasone can be used. One reason for using naturally occurring steroids is their intrinsic mineralocorticoid activity, and some patients do well on hydrocortisone alone, although most with primary AI require the addition of a synthetic mineralocorticoid such as fludrocortisone (aldosterone itself is degraded after oral administration and is therefore ineffective).

A patient with adrenal insufficiency must increase his or her glucocorticoid dose (not the mineralocorticoid) during severe stress (e.g., illness or surgery). Failure to do so may result in hospitalization and even death.

Inborn errors of cortisol biosynthesis: congenital adrenal hyperplasia

The congenital adrenal hyperplasias (CAH) are a group of autosomal recessive disorders of steroid biosynthesis. There are several different types, depending on the enzymatic block. The common element in each is that an end product is not made, leading to increase in ACTH and hence adrenal hyperplasia. The clinical findings seen depend on the enzyme defect and the precursor that accumulates. Problems seen include virilization (increased androgens and precursors), feminization (decreased androgens), adrenal insufficiency (decreased glucocorticoids), and/or hypertension (increased mineralocorticoid precursors). A vicious cycle is produced in which inadequate formation of an end product (e.g., cortisol) leads to increased ACTH and accumulation of precursors (e.g., androgen) since the desired product cannot be made adequately.

The most common type of CAH is 21α-hydroxylase deficiency. In this disorder, the enzymatic block leads to inadequate aldosterone and cortisol production, and adrenal crisis and shock shortly after birth if untreated. Instead, androgenic precursors accumulate, resulting in virilization of girls, ambiguous genitalia, and a disorder of sexual differentiation or 46, XX DSD (male appearance in a genetic female). It is the most common cause of ambiguous genitalia in the female. In boys, it results in virilization at an early age, causing severe psychological and developmental problems. In both sexes, early excess of sex steroids results in precocious puberty, with an initial increase in growth velocity and eventual short stature due to early fusion of the epiphyseal plates (from androgen excess; the excess androgen is then aromatized to estradiol, which is what causes plate fusion).

The goals of treatment are prevention of adrenal crisis and death, early recognition in women so that they can be reared as the correct sex, and early treatment in both sexes to prevent precocious puberty and the resultant short adult stature and psychological problems.

Other, much rarer forms include 3β-hydroxysteroid dehydrogenase deficiency, which can result in a similar picture of hirsutism and virilization in females. 11β-hydroxylase and 17α-hydroxylase deficiency result in the accumulation of mineralocorticoid precursors (such as deoxycorticosterone (DOC)) and can cause hypertension. The latter deficiency results in lack of feminization in women and lack of virilization in men, due to defects in the sex steroid synthetic pathway.

All forms of CAH are treated by administering gluco-corticoids (e.g., hydrocortisone), which decrease ACTH levels to normal and reduce synthesis of excess steroid precursors. Mineralocorticoids (fludrocortisone) may also be required in some patients.

Mineralocorticoids

Aldosterone is the primary mineralocorticoid and is produced by the zona glomerulosa layer of the adrenal cortex. The purpose of this hormone is to help the body hold on to sodium and excrete potassium, hence the name "mineralocorticoid." Unlike the inner two layers, ACTH is not necessary for its proper secretion. Instead, it is under the regulation of the renin–angiotensin system, involving the kidneys and liver. The stimulus for aldos-terone secretion begins in the kidney, which secretes the hormone renin in response to hypotension, decreased intravascular volume, increased serum osmolality, and hyperkalemia. Under the influence of renin, the hepatic peptide angiotensinogen is converted to angiotensin I. Another enzyme, angiotensin-converting enzyme, con-verts angiotensin I to angiotensin II. Angiotensin II then stimulates the zona glomerulosa to make aldosterone. Aldosterone then does its thing, by helping the body retain salt and water and excrete potassium. Once these levels return to normal, the kidney stops making renin, and all is well.

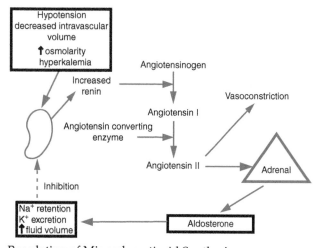

Regulation of Mineralocorticoid Synthesis

Those with secondary adrenal insufficiency (due to pituitary or hypothalamic disease) do not require a mineralocorticoid, since the aldosterone layer is not ACTH dependent. The zona glomerulosa goes on making aldosterone just fine without ACTH.

Hyperaldosteronism

Just as glucocorticoids may be secreted in excess, min-eralocorticoid hypersecretion may also occur, leading to the clinical syndrome of hyperaldosteronism. Here, excess aldosterone results in potassium loss from the kidneys, low serum potassium levels (hypokalemia), and hypertension. It is suggested by the finding of spontaneous hypokalemia (i.e., not due to drugs such as diuretics) with elevated serum and/or urinary aldos-terone levels. Primary hyperaldosteronism is due to autonomous hypersecretion from the adrenal itself, and is not dependent on the renin–angiotensin system; renin levels are therefore low. Secondary hyperaldos-teronism is due to a condition that elevates renin levels. Most commonly this is due to renovascular hypertension, but it also may be caused by a renin-secreting tumor.

Primary aldosteronism is typically (2/3 of the time) due to a benign adrenal tumor (Conn's syndrome). In most of the other cases, the hyperaldosteronism is due to enlargement (hyperplasia) of both adrenal glands. Hyperaldosteronism is rarely caused by adreno-cortical carcinoma and congenital adrenal enzyme defects. Glucocorticoid-remediable aldosteronism (GRA) is an uncommon genetic cause of hyperaldostero-nism, which results in aldosterone production by the ACTH-dependent zona fasciculata. In this rare disorder, the genes are "scrambled" so that the zona fasciculata contains aldosterone synthase and responds to ACTH stimulation (remember that normally aldosterone is regulated not by ACTH but by the renin–angiotensin system). Administration of small doses of glucocorti-coid ameliorates the hypertension and other biochemical findings.

Tumors causing hyperaldosteronism are typically excised, and the remaining adrenal is adequate for the rest of the body's needs. Hypokalemia usually resolves, and the hypertension improves. Since "incidental" adrenal tumors are quite common, it is essential to be sure that an adrenal mass, if found, is actually the cause (and not present coincidentally in a patient with hyperplasia). Adrenal vein sampling is often done to verify this; a "step-up" gradient in aldosterone is seen in the affected gland, but left and right sides show similar values in hyperplasia.

Hyperaldosteronism due to bilateral hyperplasia ("idiopathic" hyperaldosteronism) is best treated with medication, since removal of both adrenal glands, inter-estingly, does not help the hypertension (and carries significant morbidity as the patient would then require lifetime steroid replacement). A very rare cause of hyperaldosteronism is adrenocortical carcinoma, which typically carries a poor prognosis.

Occasionally, ingestion of certain substances can mimic hyperaldosteronism. True confectionary licorice (not commonly available in the United States, as candies and such merely contain licorice flavoring) and some other items (e.g., chewing tobacco, herbal preparations) contain a steroid (glycyrrhetinic acid) that inhibits an enzyme needed for conversion of cortisol to cortisone in the kidneys. Remember that cortisol has mineralocorticoid activity; if glycyrrhetinic acid inhibits degradation of cortisol in the kidney, it can overwhelm the receptor and create a form of apparent mineralocorticoid excess, causing hypertension and hypokalemia. The hypertension abates after discontinuation of the offending substance.

Cardiac hormones and sodium metabolism

In addition to antidiuretic hormone and mineralocorticoids, there are other factors that influence sodium excretion. It was discovered long ago that distention of the atrium resulted in increased water excretion. Later it was discovered that a peptide hormone, atrial natriuretic peptide (ANP), is secreted by cardiac atrial cells. Volume overload causes atrial distention, resulting in release of ANP. ANP primarily affects the kidney, where it results in natriuresis, increased glomerular filtration rate, and decreased renin secretion. It also inhibits adrenal cortical aldosterone production.

Renovascular hypertension (renal artery stenosis)

Renal artery stenosis is a relatively common condition and is often caused by atherosclerotic disease. These lesions result in stenosis and decreased blood flow to the kidneys. This fools the kidneys into thinking that blood pressure is low, and tricks them into producing more renin. This in turn produces more angiotensin II and aldosterone, resulting in hypertension (a form of "secondary" aldosteronism). Despite the increased blood pressure, the kidneys still think that the blood pressure is low (due to the stenotic lesions). This vicious cycle results in hypertension.

This type of hypertension should be considered in any person under age 25 or over 55 who develops hypertension. It may be corrected with angioplasty (inflating a balloon across the stenotic lesion) or by surgically correcting the stenotic artery.

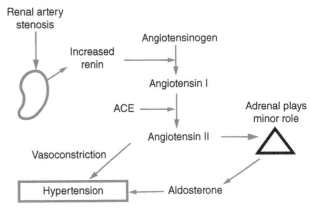

Renovascular Hypertension

ADRENAL MEDULLA

For our purposes, we will consider the adrenal medulla a separate entity from the adrenal cortex. The medulla is responsible for secreting catecholamines (epinephrine, norepinephrine, and dopamine), which are made from the amino acid tyrosine. The same types of cells are also found in the central nervous system and in the sympathetic chain. The major catecholamine secreted by the medulla is epinephrine (adrenaline). Norepinephrine is more abundant in extramedullary tissues.

There are no well-defined trophic hormones for the adrenal medulla. The catecholamines tend to increase when the body experiences physical or mental stress. This is the well-described fight-or-flight response, with increase in heart rate and other hormones (cortisol and growth hormone).

Catecholamine excess is seen in the syndrome of pheochromocytoma, discussed below. Hypofunction of the adrenal medulla is seldom clinically significant, since catecholamines are made in other sites of the body (e.g., sympathetic nervous chain). Patients with longstanding diabetes may develop autonomic neuropathy and lack of catecholamine response to hypoglycemia (hypoglycemia unawareness); this is a serious complication that can significantly impair daily life.

Catecholamine excess: pheochromocytoma

Pheochromocytoma is a neuroendocrine tumor that produces excess catecholamines. It is usually a benign tumor, but can be malignant in rare cases. Most "pheos" occur within the adrenal medulla itself. It was once felt to be an uncommon cause of hypertension, and for this reason it is sometimes a missed diagnosis. But, in fact, it can be the cause of hypertension in up to 0.6% of hypertensives. Although we all have occasional bursts of catecholamine excess when we are upset or are under stress, those with pheochromocytoma have it most of the time. During these severe episodes ("paroxysms") of excess, patients have numerous symptoms, such as diaphoresis, headache, tachycardia, pallor, and severe hypertension. These symptoms can be so severe that the patient dies of a stroke or myocardial infarction.

Pheochromocytoma may be diagnosed by several methods. The most common method is to measure catecholamines or their metabolites (metanephrines and vanillylmandelic acid (VMA)) in urine collected for a 24-h period. "Spot" urine collections are less useful. The measurement of plasma-free metanephrines has been found to have the greatest sensitivity (99%) and specificity (90%) for pheochromocytoma, compared to 80–90% for urine catecholamines. After the presence of pheochromocytoma has been confirmed biochemically, localization studies (MRI or CT) should be done.

The treatment for most tumors is surgical excision. The patient must first be prepared with α-blocking agents (phenoxybenzamine), which help control the blood pressure. After adequate α-blockade has occurred, the heart rate may be slowed with β-blockers (propranolol). Starting the β-blocker first can actually make the condition worse, so this must be avoided.

Pheochromocytoma most commonly occurs sporadically, but can also occur as part of several genetic syndromes. It was once felt that only 10% were genetically determined, but today we know that at least 20% are part of a specific genetic disorder. (The old pheochromocytoma maxim "10% extra-adrenal, 10% bilateral, 10% malignant" no longer holds true.) These syndromes also can include paragangliomas (rare neuroendocrine tumors that arise from the extra-adrenal autonomic paraganglia, derived from the neural crest). Genetic pheochromocytoma–paraganglioma syndromes include multiple endocrine neoplasia (MEN) 2, von Hippel–Lindau disease (VHL), familial paraganglioma syndromes (due to mutations in the succinate dehydrogenase (SD) genes), and neurofibromatosis (NF). Genetic markers are available for these syndromes.

INCIDENTAL ADRENAL TUMORS

An incidentally found adrenal tumor (incidentaloma) is a mass ≥1 cm in diameter that is accidentally discovered while doing another imaging modality. A common clinical scenario: a patient in an automobile crash who undergoes an abdominal CT in the emergency department is found to have an unexpected adrenal mass.

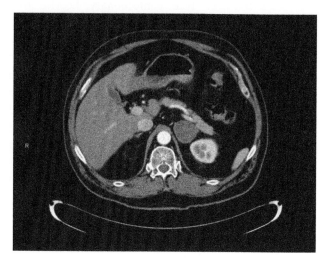

Left Adrenal Mass Found Incidentally on CT Scan

Adrenal incidentalomas are quite common (2–4% of normal adults); these masses most commonly represent benign nonfunctional cortical adenomas, but can also be functional adenomas, carcinomas, pheochromocytomas, cysts, or, rarely, metastases from other primary tumors. So, while most are of no clinical significance, they cannot simply be ignored. The challenge lies in evaluating these in a cost-effective manner without exposing the patient to needless testing or procedures.

Fortunately, certain imaging characteristics of CT are very useful in their evaluation. Lesions with low density (<10 Hounsfield units (HU), an indication of radiodensity) are usually benign (as they are lipid rich), as are those that wash out greater than 50% of radiocontrast at 15 min. Pheochromocytomas and adrenal cortical carcinomas are generally larger and have higher density (typically >40 HU).

However, even a benign-appearing lesion should be evaluated for hyperfunction, as hormonal excess can have insidious, harmful effects. This generally includes an evaluation for Cushing's syndrome and pheochromocytoma. Hyperaldosteronism should be excluded in patients with hypertension and hypokalemia (although aldosterone-producing tumors are often quite small and not discovered incidentally).

Functional tumors should be removed. Those with benign radiologic appearance who are deemed nonfunctional (most incidentalomas fall into this category) can be simply monitored with periodic biochemical screening and CT scans. Lesions > 6 cm in diameter should be removed, regardless of the biochemistry. Those that are 4–6 cm are of "intermediate risk" and may require surgical excision, depending on the individual situation. Obviously, significant interval growth of a lesion is usually a reason to remove it.

REVIEW QUESTIONS

1. A 47-year-old overweight woman undergoes an abdominal CT with contrast after presenting to the ED with severe abdominal pain. A 1.5 cm low-density left adrenal mass (5 HU) is seen, with 60% washout of contrast at 15 min. She has a history of hypertension and type 2 diabetes, for which she takes lisinopril, metformin, and sitagliptin. Her examination is normal except for her weight.
   a. What common abnormality are we concerned about here?
   b. How would we evaluate this?
   c. Are her diabetes and hypertension likely linked to it?
   (a) She has an incidentally discovered adrenal mass, common in adults (2–4%).
   (b) The appearance on CT is that of a benign adenoma, but hyperfunction must be excluded. An overnight dexamethasone suppression test was done, and was normal. Even though the appearance is not consistent with a pheochromocytoma, plasma catecholamines and metanephrines were normal.
   (c) Likely not. Millions of people have hypertension and diabetes, and very few cases are explainable by an endocrine problem. Cushing's syndrome should be excluded, but is statistically unlikely.

2. A 42-year-old woman presents with muscle weakness (unable to climb a flight of stairs), colored abdominal striae, central obesity, new onset hypertension and diabetes mellitus, and depression over the last 18 months. She is a nonsmoker and takes no medications except for a multivitamin. Serum cortisol after 1 mg overnight dexamethasone suppression is elevated at 7.7 µg/dL (normal: <2 µg/dL); serum ACTH is three times the upper limit of normal. The most likely diagnosis is:
   a. Cushing's syndrome due to functioning adrenocortical adenoma
   b. Cushing's syndrome due to functioning adrenocortical carcinoma
   c. Factitious abuse of corticosteroids
   d. Cushing's disease due to ACTH-secreting pituitary adenoma
   e. Cushing's syndrome due to small cell lung carcinoma
   (d) This is a classic presentation of Cushing's disease, the most common (2/3 of cases) cause of endogenous Cushing's syndrome (CS). Functioning adrenal tumors (a, b) and exogenous steroids (c) are excluded due to the elevated ACTH level (in these disorders, it should be suppressed). While ectopic ACTH syndrome (e) is theoretically possible, it usually presents much more rapidly; this woman is also not of a demographic group at high risk for lung cancer. A pituitary MRI should be done at this time after a second test confirms the presence of CS.

3. A 19-year-old Caucasian college student presents to an emergency department in Minneapolis, MN, with a 6-week history of weight loss, anorexia, nausea, and vomiting. She is hypotensive and noted to be diffusely hyperpigmented (it is January; she denies recent travel to warm climates or tanning booth usage). Serum chemistries are remarkable for hyperkalemia and hyponatremia. Random serum cortisol is 2.2 µg/dL; 1 h after administration of synthetic ACTH, serum cortisol is 6.2 µg/dL (normal response: >18 µg/dL). Serum pregnancy test is negative; ACTH level is pending. The most appropriate next step in her management is:
   a. Adrenal CT imaging
   b. Pituitary MRI
   c. Measurement of pituitary hormones (growth hormone, prolactin, FSH, LH, TSH)
   d. Administration of intravenous saline and hydrocortisone
   e. Dexamethasone suppression test
   (d) This young woman has a classic presentation of Addison's disease (primary adrenocortical insufficiency). The presence of these symptoms plus hyperpigmentation during the winter in a cold-climate

area without evidence of UV exposure is strongly suggestive of this diagnosis; the lack of response to synthetic ACTH confirms the diagnosis. The ACTH level should be grossly elevated when the result returns from the lab. Adrenal CT (a) might be necessary in certain indications (e.g., when infections or malignancy-associated etiologies are suspected), but is not generally needed in such a typical presentation, which is usually autoimmune-mediated. Pituitary MRI would not be indicated. Pituitary hormone measurement (c) would not be helpful (although TSH might be measured, as some patients also have coexistent hypothyroidism). A dexamethasone suppression test (e) is used for the diagnosis of Cushing's syndrome (cortisol excess), not deficiency.

4. A 21-year-old male college student presents with new onset hypertension with significant hypokalemia. He has been trying to quit smoking and instead has taken up chewing tobacco; the particular brand he has been using is noted to contain *Glycyrrhiza uralensis* root (licorice) as a sweetener. He was normotensive 1 year ago when he went to the student health center for an upper respiratory infection. The next best step in management would be:

    a. Measurement of serum aldosterone and renin levels

    b. Adrenal CT to search for an aldosterone-producing tumor

    c. Renal angiogram to search for renal artery stenosis

    d. Discontinuation of chewing tobacco

    e. Start antihypertensive medication

    (d) This is a typical case of inadvertent ingestion of glycyrrhetic acid, the active ingredient in licorice, which inhibits the enzyme 11-β-hydroxysteroid dehydrogenase that normally metabolizes the active cortisol to inactive cortisone in the kidney; given sufficient enzyme inhibition, cortisol levels in the kidney can reach levels that can cause apparent mineralocorticoid excess. Licorice is an FDA-approved food supplement found in a number of readily available preparations, without regulations to prevent toxicity. (Common licorice-flavored candies in the United States do not contain glycyrrhetic acid.) This case illustrates the need to take a careful medical history before pursuing an expensive and unrewarding workup for unlikely disorders in this age patient.

5. A 62-year-old male patient presents to the emergency department with severe headaches, palpitations, tremors, and "fear of impending doom." He was recently started on atenolol (a β-blocker) by his primary physician for the hypertension, which has made the episodes worse. Prior to this there was no history of hypertension. His laboratory evaluation has included a normal 24-h urinary free cortisol, normal electrolytes and chemistry panel. A 24-h urine for catecholamines and metanephrines is notable for significant elevation of norepinephrine and normetanephrine; plasma normetanephrine is eight times the normal upper limit. Abdominal CT in the emergency department reveals a 3-cm left adrenal mass with density of 40 HU. In addition to admission to the hospital for monitoring, the most appropriate management of this patient at this time includes:

    a. Increasing the dose of the β-blocker

    b. Immediate resection of the adrenal mass

    c. Observation and repeat CT in 6 months

    d. Prompt discontinuation of atenolol, and administration of α-blockade to control hypertension, then re-initiating β-blockade after that, followed by surgical removal

    e. Fine needle aspiration biopsy of the adrenal mass, as the high Hounsfield density likely indicates an adrenocortical malignancy

    (d) This is a classic presentation of pheochromocytoma. Hypertension presenting in a person this age must raise flags for a secondary cause; pheochromocytoma is more common than previously thought. The CT appearance is typical for this type of tumor; while adrenocortical adenomas are low density (<10 HU), pheochromocytomas are very vascular and more dense. While carcinomas (e) also are of higher density, the clinical picture is typical of pheochromocytoma. Biopsy of the tumor is not indicated and could lead to catastrophic consequences (and even death); immediate resection of the mass (b) would be similarly haphazard.

    A common presentation is the "unmasking" of symptoms by prescription of a β-blocker; unopposed β-blockade in pheochromocytoma can paradoxically worsen the condition. Therefore, increasing the dose of atenolol (a) is contraindicated. The proper management is α-blockade (phenoxybenzamine) followed by β-blockade (after the hypertension has been controlled) and surgical resection. Observation (c) is a bad idea, as this disorder has a very high mortality rate if untreated.

6. A 78-year-old female patient with history of chronic dementia and rheumatoid arthritis is admitted to the hospital for pneumonia. Shortly after admission, she is noted to be hypotensive and mildly hyponatremic. Her skin is pale; she does not answer questions coherently, consistent with her prior mental state. Serum cortisol is very low, and does not respond to challenge with synthetic ACTH; plasma ACTH is also suppressed. ECG and cardiac markers of ischemia are negative. What is the most likely cause of her decompensation?
   a. She has developed primary adrenal insufficiency due to antibiotics given for pneumonia
   b. She was on prednisone at the nursing home for rheumatoid arthritis, and this was inadvertently missed from her medication list when she was admitted to the hospital
   c. She has developed an acute decompensation of her dementia
   d. She is on a medication that is interfering with the cortisol assay, leading to falsely decreased values

(b) This is a classic presentation of secondary adrenal insufficiency, usually due to abrupt discontinuation of steroids. Even small doses of prednisone (e.g., 5 mg daily) are enough to cause adrenal suppression and insufficiency if withdrawn. This patient should receive stress steroid doses while in the hospital; it is imperative to carefully review all patient records on admission (especially in a demented patient who cannot give a coherent history) so that such errors can be avoided.

LECTURE 5 — Glucose Metabolism

REVIEW

In the last lecture we learned about the adrenal glands, which are also called the "fight-or-flight" glands. These glands secrete hormones that are necessary during physical stress and illness and are required for life.

The two adrenal glands lie in the retroperitoneal cavity above the kidneys. The adrenal is divided into the outer adrenal cortex and the inner medulla. The adrenal cortex contains three layers that make steroid hormones. The steroids made by the adrenals include glucocorticoids, sex steroids, and mineralocorticoids. Sex steroid secretion is minimal when compared to those derived from the gonads.

Glucocorticoids are essential to life. They are called this because they increase glucose concentrations by increasing gluconeogenesis. The trophic hormone for glucocorticoid synthesis is the pituitary hormone ACTH—ACTH stimulation results in increased glucocorticoid synthesis, and decreased ACTH results in deficiency. The primary glucocorticoid of interest is cortisol (hydrocortisone).

Cushing's syndrome is a condition of cortisol excess. It may be caused by ACTH hypersecretion or be ACTH independent in nature. The most common cause of Cushing's syndrome is called Cushing's disease, a condition resulting from a pituitary tumor that secretes too much ACTH. Cushing's syndrome may also be caused by non-adrenal tumors that secrete ACTH. This is called ectopic ACTH syndrome. ACTH-independent causes of Cushing's syndrome include adrenal tumors and endogenous steroid ingestion. Clinical features of Cushing's syndrome include muscle weakness, excessive bruising, pigmented striae, central obesity, and a "moon face."

Adrenal insufficiency is the opposite of Cushing's syndrome, and may be caused by a variety of conditions.

Primary adrenal insufficiency (Addison's disease) usually results from autoimmune destruction of the adrenal gland, but can also be caused by infiltrative diseases or infectious causes such as tuberculosis or fungal infections. Secondary adrenal insufficiency may be caused by hypopituitarism; patients who have been receiving exogenous glucocorticoids may also develop secondary adrenal insufficiency after the drugs are withdrawn too quickly.

Patients with Addison's disease have elevated ACTH levels, since this is a primary organ deficiency syndrome. This increased ACTH often results in a hyperpigmented appearance because of the biochemical similarity of ACTH to melanocyte-stimulating hormone (MSH), important in lower animals. Other signs and symptoms of adrenal insufficiency include anorexia, weakness, hypotension, hypoglycemia, and hyperkalemia. Adrenal insufficiency is easily treated with oral glucocorticoids.

The congenital adrenal hyperplasias (CAH) are a group of inherited disorders of steroid biosynthesis. These disorders may result in problems due to (1) inadequate production of necessary steroids (e.g., cortisol) or (2) accumulation of steroid precursors with undesirable properties (e.g., androgens). The most common form is 21-hydroxylase deficiency, which may lead to masculinization of women and early virilization of men, and precocious puberty and short stature in both genders.

Mineralocorticoids are also made by the adrenal cortex. Aldosterone is the primary mineralocorticoid of interest and its synthesis is regulated by the renin–angiotensin system, not the pituitary gland. Patients with primary adrenal insufficiency have mineralocorticoid deficiency and require replacement. Hypopituitarism therefore does not result in significant mineralocorticoid deficiency, and patients with secondary adrenal insufficiency do not require mineralocorticoid replacement.

Aldosterone excess results in hyperaldosteronism. This in turn results in hypokalemia due to increased potassium excretion by the kidneys. Severe hypertension may also result. The most common cause of hyperaldosteronism is an adrenal tumor (benign or malignant). Treatment is surgical excision of the tumor. Most other cases of hyperaldosteronism are caused by bilateral hyperplasia, and these patients are best managed medically (with aldosterone antagonists such as spironolactone and eplerenone).

Renovascular hypertension is a relatively common cause of hypertension. This is caused by stenosis (blockage) of the renal artery, which fools the kidney into thinking that decreased blood flow is present. The kidney therefore tells the liver to produce more angiotensin II, resulting in a form of secondary hyperaldosteronism. This may be treated by correction of the stenotic lesion.

Finally, the adrenal medulla is important in the synthesis of catecholamines. Catecholamines are also synthesized in other neural tissues. A disorder of clinical interest in the adrenal medulla is pheochromocytoma, which produces excess catecholamines and results in severe hypertension, stroke, and even death. These tumors are typically benign and usually unilateral, although bilateral tumors may occur; they are being increasingly recognized as a part of certain genetic syndromes. They are best treated by surgical excision after proper patient preparation with α- and β-blockade.

GLUCOSE METABOLISM

All living organisms require energy to survive. We obtain energy by ingesting fuels such as carbohydrates, protein, and lipids. This is called the anabolic (building) phase of energy metabolism. The body may also synthesize carbohydrates and lipids as needed. In the well-fed state, excess glucose is converted to glycogen, a compound made of multiple glucose molecules linked together. After the glycogen stores are filled, excess glucose is used for fatty acid synthesis. Glucose is to some extent like the "team manager" for our football team; it is not glamorous, but it provides the energy necessary for functions of the rest of the body; like the team manager, when the system malfunctions, the consequences can be severe.

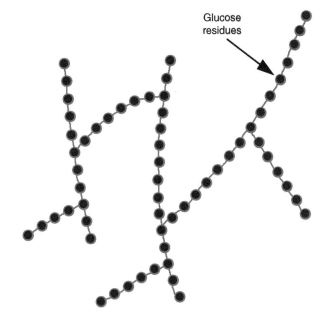

Glucose residues

Glycogen

CH2OH

Glucose

Problems result when disequilibrium between these two phases occurs. The risk of an inadequate anabolic phase (eating too little) is starvation and death, while excess anabolism (eating too much) results in energy excess and obesity. Obesity can only occur when energy expended is less than energy taken in. Overweight persons who declare they "eat hardly anything" would be violating fundamental laws of physics that state that (1) matter can neither be created nor destroyed and that (2) energy is proportional to mass. It is true, though, that many overweight persons have a low basal metabolic rate and do not expend much energy, making it difficult for them to lose weight. However, while some folks have a different metabolic rate than others, it is hard to become overweight without eating too much.

The catabolic or breakdown state is necessary to maintain energy levels 4–6 h after eating. The body's immediate energy needs can be met by glycogen breakdown to glucose. Glycogen stores, however, only last about 12 h after fasting and cannot meet long-term energy needs. After that, fatty acid oxidation is required.

In this lecture, we will discuss the common disorders of glucose metabolism, such as diabetes mellitus.

Insulin and glucagon

Understanding insulin's effects is important in the study of glucose metabolism. Insulin is a protein hormone produced in the β (beta) cells of the pancreas. Insulin starts out as the precursor molecule preproinsulin, which is then cleaved to proinsulin in the cell. Proinsulin is next broken up into insulin and C-peptide (connecting peptide); the latter historically has been felt to have no biological activity, although some have postulated that it may be of some clinical significance.

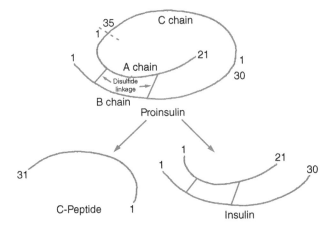

Proinsulin and Cleavage Products

Insulin is an anabolic hormone that promotes energy storage. It promotes glycogen and fatty acid synthesis, glycolysis, and triglyceride storage, and inhibits glycogenolysis, hepatic ketogenesis, and gluconeogenesis. Insulin increases glucose transport across cell membranes by means of glucose transporters (GLUTs). Many different GLUTs have been identified; for example, GLUT-4 is found in muscle and adipose tissue; GLUT-3 is found in neurons. Insulin levels rise in response to a sugar load and decrease when levels return to normal. A basal amount of insulin is always necessary for maintenance of glucose homeostasis, even in the fasting state.

Glucagon is made in the α (alpha) cells of the pancreas, and is sort of an antagonist to insulin. Its function is catabolic (it breaks down molecules to provide energy for cells), in contrast to insulin, which is anabolic in nature (builds molecules). Secretion is inhibited by high glucose and fatty acid levels, and stimulated by hypoglycemia. It is very important in recovery from hypoglycemia, and many diabetic patients develop a loss of glucagon response to hypoglycemia (via the same inflammatory process that destroyed the β cells). These patients keep injectable glucagon on hand for use in cases of severe hypoglycemia. The pancreatic hormone somatostatin (also made in the hypothalamus) inhibits secretion of both glucagon and insulin.

Amylin (human islet amyloid polypeptide, IAPP) also plays a role in glycemic regulation by slowing gastric emptying and promoting satiety, thereby preventing postprandial spikes in blood glucose levels. The secretion of IAPP diminishes in type 1 diabetes, and new drugs designed to replace this have shown promise in certain individuals; these will be discussed later.

Diabetes mellitus

Diabetes mellitus (DM) is a disorder of glucose metabolism whose name is derived from the Greek words diabetes ("siphon") and mellitus ("sweet"), and was first described in an Egyptian papyrus dated 1500 B.C. Ancient civilizations noted that ants were attracted to the high-glucose urine of patients with diabetes. Early medical practitioners also made a distinction between two types of diabetes. The first form occurred in children and young adults who were thin; these individuals essentially "wasted away" and died within a few years. This type of diabetes results from absence or deficiency of insulin and is called type 1 diabetes. Another, more indolent, form was described in older, overweight individuals (although fewer people were overweight then than today). This is called type 2 diabetes and is caused by impaired insulin action (insulin resistance).

Diabetes Mellitus Classification

Type 1 DM	Requires insulin for life; ketoacidosis and death occur without insulin. May develop at all ages but more common in children, adolescents, and young adults. Mostly immune mediated
Type 2 DM	End result of insulin resistance, leading to inefficient use of insulin. Insulin deficiency may occur later in the disease. Patients are often (but not always) overweight, and may require insulin for control (although they are ketosis resistant)
Gestational DM	DM specifically diagnosed during pregnancy, caused by the anti-insulin properties of human chorionic somatomammotropin, a placental hormone. Must be distinguished from preexisting DM in those who become pregnant. True GDM generally abates after delivery
Other	DM caused by other conditions (e.g., cystic fibrosis, chronic pancreatitis, pancreatectomy, hemochromatosis, Cushing's syndrome) or medications (e.g., antiretroviral drugs, glucocorticoids)

Diabetes is an extremely common disorder, affecting approximately 5% of the US population. In the United States, type 2 is much more common, accounting for 90% of those with diabetes. The prevalence of type 2 has increased as obesity and sedentary lifestyles have become more common; indeed, the incidence of type 2 diabetes in adolescents has been increasing at an alarming rate; the percentage of type 2 DM in pediatric patients with diabetes in 1990 was only 3%, but rose to 20% by the mid-2000s and is expected to continue increasing.

The remaining 10% of diabetic patients have type 1 diabetes. This type is more common in those of northern European descent (e.g., Sweden and Finland), and less common in those of African, Asian, or Hispanic descent. Whatever the classification, diabetes is an enormous economic problem—the estimated cost of diabetes and its complications is one out of every seven health care dollars.

Patients with diabetes cannot use glucose effectively, resulting in hyperglycemia. A large load of glucose is filtered through to the kidney, carrying water with it; this results in the typical symptom of excessive urination (polyuria). Since the body loses too much water, excessive thirst (polydipsia) occurs. Finally, since the body cannot use glucose properly, it thinks it is in a starved state, and excessive eating (polyphagia) occurs. The body also breaks down fats and proteins in an effort to compensate for decreased energy utilization (which is not very efficient). In essence, then, the body is starved for fuel despite having too much of it! These three symptoms are called the "classic symptoms" of diabetes or "polys." Not all patients with diabetes have symptoms, however; many persons with type 2 diabetes are asymptomatic for years before diabetes is discovered on a routine screening test.

There are four accepted ways to diagnose diabetes (of any type): (1) two fasting serum glucose levels $\geq 126\,mg/dL$ (7.0 mmol/L); (2) serum glucose level $\geq 200\,mg/dL$ (11.1 mmol/L) 2h after a 75 g glucose load; (3) classic symptoms of diabetes with serum glucose $\geq 200\,mg/dL$; (4) hemoglobin A_{1c} (HbA$_{1c}$) level $\geq 6.5\,mg/dL$. For all criteria except (3), when the diagnosis of diabetes is obvious, the test should be repeated with a confirmatory test, given the enormous psychological and potential economic cost to the patient who is given a diagnosis of diabetes.

Impaired glucose tolerance is a term used to describe those whose glucose levels are not entirely normal but who do not meet the criteria above. They are in a "gray area" between normal and diabetic and were once called "borderline diabetics," an outdated term; "prediabetes" is more appropriate today. To many patients, such a term implies (erroneously) that the condition is neither important nor serious, while it is certainly a condition that warrants monitoring. Impaired fasting glucose is a similar term, given to those with a serum glucose value between 100 and 126 mg/dL (5.5–7.0 mmol/L).

Type 1 diabetes

This type is also called insulin-dependent diabetes mellitus (IDDM), and results from the near-total deficiency of insulin. (While some type 2 patients require insulin for glucose control, they do not typically die of acute complications without it, so they are more properly

Diagnostic Criteria for Diabetes (Excludes Gestational DM)

Measurement	Normal	Prediabetes (Impaired Glucose Tolerance)	Diabetes	Remarks
Fasting glucose	<100 mg/dL (5.5 mmol/L)	100–125 mg/dL (5.5–6.9 mmol/L)	≥126 mg/dL (7.0 mmol/L)	Should be repeated to confirm
Oral glucose tolerance test (OGTT) (75 g), 2 h value	<140 mg/dL (7.7 mmol/L)	140–199 mg/dL (7.7–10.9 mmol/L)	≥200 mg/dL (11.0 mmol/L)	Intermediate (30 min and 1 h) values can be used to screen for prediabetes (impaired glucose tolerance); should be repeated to confirm
Random glucose measurement	n/a	n/a	≥200 mg/dL (11.0 mmol/L)	Must be accompanied by classic symptoms (polyuria, polydipsia)
Hemoglobin A_{1c}	<5.7%	5.7–6.4%	≥6.5%	Should be repeated to confirm; must conform to certain laboratory standards

termed "insulin-requiring.") Type 1 DM was once called "juvenile diabetes," but this archaic term is not at all accurate because, although it is more common in children and young adults, it may develop in older adults (even those in their sixth or seventh decade of life). And, as we will discuss later, type 2 diabetes may also occur in younger individuals (the age of onset is decreasing due to more children and young adults being overweight or obese).

Type 1 DM is typically an autoimmune disease, resulting in destruction of pancreatic islet cells by anti-islet cell antibodies (ILA) with the presence of antibodies against glutamic acid decarboxylase (GAD) and other islet cell targets. Deficiency of insulin results in hyperglycemia, ketoacidosis, and death if untreated.

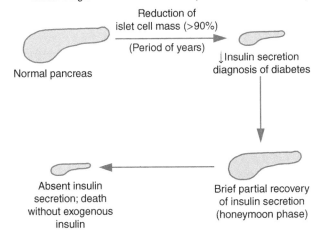

Type 1 (Insulin Dependent) Diabetes

The typical patient with type 1 DM is a patient presenting with a several week period of weight loss, polyuria, polydipsia, and polyphagia. If this process continues without medical intervention, ketoacidosis (and eventually death) will result. Indeed, before the discovery of insulin (early 1920s) this disorder was a death sentence, and life could only be prolonged a brief time. Prompt initiation of insulin therapy is necessary. As mentioned above, type 1 can occur in older adults, although type 2 is more common in this age group. A variant of type 1 occurring in adults is called latent autoimmune diabetes in adults (LADA). These are typically thin adults who respond poorly to oral therapy and require insulin. But remember that type 1 can occur in patients of any age.

After initial diagnosis, some insulin is still present in most new type 1 patients, and a brief state of remission often occurs in which symptoms and glucose levels appear to normalize. This "honeymoon phase" is short-lived (typically several months, but can be longer) followed by absolute dependence on exogenous insulin to sustain life.

Like all autoimmune diseases, type 1 diabetes appears to require both a genetic predisposition and an environmental trigger. Those with certain genetic (human leukocyte antigen or HLA) markers are predisposed to develop type 1 diabetes; the disorder is most common in those of northern European descent. But this alone is not enough—the (as yet unidentified) environmental insult must also occur. For example, if one identical twin develops type 1 diabetes, the chance of the remaining twin developing it is only about 50%. If the second twin develops it, it may be much later in life than the first twin. This is in contrast to type 2 diabetes, where over 98% of second identical twins develop the disorder.

The autoimmune form of type 1 diabetes is the most common form of type 1 and is sometimes called type 1A diabetes. Individuals with type 1B diabetes have a similar clinical manifestation but seem to lack the autoantibodies present in type 1A. A majority of patients with the non-autoimmune form of type 1 are of African-American or Asian racial backgrounds; type 2 diabetes is much more common in these ethnic groups.

Patients who have undergone a pancreatectomy (e.g., for malignancy) or in whom the β cells are destroyed (cystic fibrosis, chronic pancreatitis, etc.) also require insulin for life. This will be discussed further under "secondary diabetes."

Type 2 diabetes

This is the more common form of diabetes (90% of patients in the United States) and is often called non-insulin dependent diabetes (NIDDM) or adult-onset diabetes. The latter term may be misleading and its use discouraged, since type 2 can also occur in children, adolescents, or young adults. Indeed, the incidence of type 2 in these younger persons is increasing as our society becomes more sedentary and overweight (20% of diabetes in the pediatric population is now type 2). A special, uncommon group of type 2 diabetes disorders called maturity-onset diabetes of the young (MODY) may occur in young people. This is distinguished from typical type 2 diabetes in that MODY is usually inherited in an autosomal dominant manner and the typical patient has several first-degree relatives with ketosis-resistant diabetes that developed at a young age; MODY may present in infancy, childhood, or adolescence. The MODY forms of diabetes are due to several different specific genetic mutations (glucokinase, hepatocyte nuclear factor 1α, etc.). However, monogenic types of diabetes such as MODY may be more common (about 2% of patients with DM) than previously thought. But, since genetic testing is expensive (>$1,000 per gene), patients undergoing genetic testing should be tested only after investigating the family history thoroughly to decide if a potential MODY phenotype exists. Remember that taking a thorough medical history does not cost extra!

Unlike type 1, which is a state of insulin deficiency, type 2 is a state of hormone resistance in which insulin receptors lose their sensitivity to insulin. Insulin secretion initially is normal; in fact, insulin levels are often elevated early in the disorder, leading to hyperinsulinism. It is like having a big car with an eight-cylinder engine with six of the spark plugs gone. The engine works very hard and burns a lot of gas, but does not propel the car very fast because of gross inefficiency. This is in contrast to type 1, which is like a car with no gas. The end result is similar (the car does not run properly), but the pathophysiology is vastly different. Many patients with type 2 are asymptomatic at the time of diagnosis and are diagnosed by routine screening.

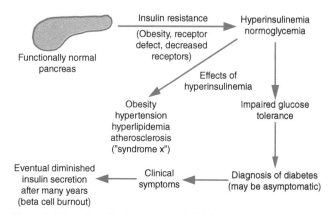

Type 2 (Non-Insulin Dependent) Diabetes

Many (but not all) patients are overweight, which accounts for the insulin resistance. Populations that are traditionally lean (e.g., Asians) are more likely to develop the disease if they move to the United States and consume a typical high-calorie Western diet. About 15% of patients, however, are of normal body weight. Type 2 DM is therefore an extremely heterogeneous disorder, with patients of all body shapes and sizes. (Type 1 patients can be obese, too, although the obesity does not cause the disorder (but may impair efforts at control).)

The evolutionary theory of natural selection postulates that deleterious genes are removed from the population because these persons die sooner and are less likely to reproduce. If this is true, then why is type 2 diabetes so common? Why would the genetics for such an undesirable disorder have survived? We might theorize that at some point in time the tendency for type 2 might actually be advantageous. How could that be? Well, for most of our years of civilization, food was not plentiful for the average person—life was hard and physically exhausting. Only the very wealthy had the luxuries of excess food and avoidance of physical labor. We know that many patients with type 2 diabetes are obese and gain weight easily with little food intake. Therefore, these people might actually have had an evolutionary advantage in a society where food was scarce and activity level high.

Food, however, is abundant in most developed countries today, and this has made the tendency for type 2 disadvantageous (genetics have not had a time to catch up). Physical activity has also diminished from our early years of civilization, contributing to obesity.

Many patients with type 2 diabetes are puzzled as to why their fasting glucose is often high in the morning. After all, they did not eat anything all night, so how could the morning glucose be high? This is explained by realizing that a cardinal derangement in type 2 diabetes is the presence of increased hepatic gluconeogenesis. Increased growth hormone secretion at night (the dawn phenomenon) also increases insulin resistance and contributes to fasting hyperglycemia. This is why many patients with type 2 benefit from an evening injection of insulin.

The tendency for type 2 DM appears to be inherited, but is not localized to specific chromosomal areas as is type 1 DM. The second, postulated environmental trigger is not necessary (since type 2 is not an autoimmune disease). The person does, however, have some control over his or her destiny, unlike in type 1 DM, where prevention trials have been disappointing. Normalization of body weight early in life leads to less risk for diabetes. Genetic penetrance is quite high with type 2. If one identical twin has NIDDM, the chance that the other will have it approaches 100%, assuming both have similar body sizes and health. In contrast, with IDDM, the likelihood of a second twin being affected is only about 50%, meaning that other (as of yet identified) nongenetic factors are necessary to develop the disorder.

Type 2 patients may exhibit a unique phenomenon called glucose toxicity. Here, the high glucose levels may actually inhibit β-cell production of insulin, creating a "vicious cycle" of hyperglycemia; improvement in β-cell function and insulin secretion results after glucose levels normalize. This phenomenon must be distinguished from the "honeymoon period" of type 1 diabetes (a temporary interval when insulin secretion returns after disease onset).

Hyperinsulinemia and metabolic syndrome

The high insulin levels in our "inefficient engine" appear to do more than just result in hyperglycemia (if that was not enough!). Hyperinsulinemia appears to result in a "vicious cycle" of metabolic problems, including atherosclerotic disease, diabetes mellitus, hypertension, and hyperlipidemia (predominantly hypertriglyceridemia).

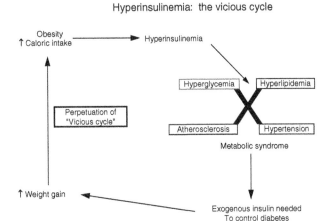

Hyperinsulinemia and Metabolic Syndrome

These problems may not all present simultaneously (e.g., a patient may experience hypertension and hypertriglyceridemia years before developing diabetes mellitus). Newer therapies for type 2 diabetes are directed at correcting the underlying problem of insulin resistance. Patients with type 2 may present for diagnosis after having already suffered many metabolic complications of their disease, because it is often asymptomatic. (The "time clock" denoting onset of disease is usually easier to specify in patients with type 1 DM, as onset is typically more abrupt.)

OBESITY

While obesity is not specifically an endocrine disease (and few endocrine disorders cause obesity, by the way), a brief discussion is in order given its importance in metabolic syndrome and diabetes.

Obesity has become a problem not only in the United States but in many other countries as well. It is a chronic, preventable, and treatable disease. Many studies have shown that an increase in body fat increases the risks of medical complications and death. As we become more sedentary, many have "paid the price" for lack of exercise and abundance of processed foods.

Obesity is a major risk factor for many diseases such as coronary artery disease, type 2 diabetes, hypertension, stroke, hyperlipidemia, venous insufficiency,

Definition of Obesity

Classification	Body Mass Index (BMI): Mass (kg)/Height^2 (m^2)
Overweight	25.0–29.9 kg/m^2
Obesity	≥30.0 kg/m^2
Class I	30.0–34.9 kg/m^2
Class II	35.0–39.9 kg/m^2
Class III	≥40 kg/m^2

osteoarthritis, steatohepatitis, cholelithiasis, and obstructive sleep apnea, among others. Unfortunately, there is no "magic bean" for obesity; if there were, such people would not exist.

The genetics for obesity, like most forms of type 2 diabetes, are heterogeneous; there are no specific markers or gene therapies available that are useful today in treating most individual patients. Specific genetic syndromes associated with obesity (e.g., Prader–Willi syndrome) do exist.

Diet and exercise is a mainstay of therapy in any patient with obesity. Remember that 1 lb (0.45 kg) of fat contains approximately 3,500 kcal of energy (1 dietary or nutritional "calorie" (as you would see on food packaging) = 1 kcal); 1 kcal is the amount of energy needed to raise the temperature of a kilogram of water by one degree Celsius. A net deficit of only 500 kcal/day will therefore result in a loss of 1 lb/week. This can be accomplished by eating 500 fewer kcal per day, expending 500 additional kcal of energy per day, or a combination of both. There is no other way to lose weight besides creating a caloric deficit (besides obvious therapies such as liposuction that physically remove adipose tissue); if you believe there is, you should brush up on your basic thermodynamics to review concepts of mass–energy conservation.

While 1 lb/week may not sound like much, it can be accomplished without too much hardship and is maintainable over the long run, unlike many "rapid weight loss" diets which are unsustainable and may even be unhealthy.

Medications may be used to treat obesity, but are often unsatisfactory. These include the short-term use of appetite suppressants such as phentermine (which has been safely used for over 50 years). The pancreatic lipase inhibitor orlistat (the only FDA-approved drug in the United States for long-term treatment of obesity) may cause modest weight loss by inhibiting intestinal absorption of fat. There are several over-the-counter preparations available, but these may actually be hazardous.

Lorcaserin is a recently introduced drug with serotonergic and anorectic properties which is approved for use in the treatment of obesity for adults with a BMI equal to or greater than 30 or adults with a BMI of 27 or greater who have at least one weight-related health condition (e.g., hypertension, type 2 diabetes, or hyperlipidemia). It has the frequent side effects of headache and sinusitis and is not meant for long-term therapy.

As a last resort, bariatric surgery is an option for morbidly obese persons. Not to be taken lightly, certain criteria should be met before consideration:

- Body mass index (BMI) 40 kg/m^2 or higher
- BMI between 35 and 40 kg/m^2, but with a serious weight-related medical problem (e.g., type 2 diabetes, hypertension, severe obstructive sleep apnea).

A team consisting of a physician, dietitian, psychologist, and bariatric surgeon will evaluate whether gastric bypass or other weight-loss surgery is the right choice for the patient; surgery is not something to be taken lightly, expense being the least of the considerations. This evaluation will help determine if the medical benefits of the patient's surgery outweigh the potentially serious risks, as this is a major surgical procedure, and complications can occur. Types of surgery include the following:

Gastric restriction alone: This is most often accomplished by gastric banding with inflatable devices whose inner circumference may be adjusted by introducing or withdrawing water from them. Gastric stapling, as with vertical banded gastroplasty, has been practically abandoned in favor of banding. The newer gastric sleeve procedure is gaining support.

Gastric restriction and intestinal malabsorption:

Roux-en-Y gastric bypass combines gastric restriction with a rerouting of stomach outflow to the latter portion of the small intestine. This intestinal bypass significantly reduces the absorptive capacity of the gut.

Biliopancreatic diversion with or without duodenal switch. This procedure reroutes the intestinal flow to bypass a good portion of the absorptive sections of the intestine, thus creating chronic malabsorption with intended weight loss. At present, the broader medical community has not been convinced that this procedure should be routinely employed.

Patients undergoing bariatric surgery require lifelong follow-up by the clinician for potential surgical complications and to monitor for long-term weight loss success. There are many considerations in selecting patients for bariatric procedures:

First, acute (surgical) complications of bariatric surgery, including leakage, can result in considerable morbidity and even death in some cases. Some (laparoscopic banding) are relatively noninvasive, but other divertive procedures are major surgeries.

Second, malabsorption of several nutrients can be a significant and variable challenge. From an endocrine perspective, the nutritional deficiencies may cause secondary hyperparathyroidism with bone mineral density loss due to calcium malabsorption, other vitamin and trace element deficiencies, and the improvement of the female gonadal axis in women with polycystic ovary syndrome (PCOS). All of these issues require ongoing involvement with these patients. Medical nutrition therapy should be modified to address these postsurgical needs.

Third, the effectiveness of the procedure can diminish over time, and weight loss or maintenance may require augmentation with lifestyle or pharmacologic interventions.

Secondary diabetes

Secondary diabetes is diabetes caused by another condition. A common secondary form is caused by repeated episodes of pancreatitis (inflammation of the pancreas), which results in reduced β-cell mass. Those who have undergone pancreatectomy obviously develop insulin deficiency and insulin-dependent diabetes. Infiltrative diseases may cause pancreatic destruction and diabetes. The most common cause is hemochromatosis, which results in excessive iron accumulation in visceral organs and pancreatic destruction. This is also called "bronze diabetes" because of the dark skin pigmentation due to iron accumulation. Drugs such as high-dose corticosteroids (e.g., prednisone) commonly cause hyperglycemia and diabetes; this condition may be reversible after discontinuation of the steroids.

Whether or not the secondary diabetes is classified as type 1 or 2 depends on the severity of the condition and extent of β cell mass lost. Once islet cell destruction exceeds 90%, insulin is almost always required.

Gestational diabetes and diabetes in pregnancy

Gestational diabetes (GDM) is yet another subset of diabetes. By definition, it develops during pregnancy (as opposed to type 1 or 2, which exist beforehand). The term usually refers to a state of reversible glucose intolerance that begins late in the second trimester of pregnancy. As the growing fetoplacental unit increases in size, substances such as human placental growth hormone and human chorionic somatomammotropin (human placental lactogen) are secreted in large amounts, and increase insulin resistance; GDM results in susceptible individuals. Risk factors include obesity, family history of type 2 diabetes, and advanced maternal age.

All pregnant women (except, of course, those who already have known diabetes) should have a GDM screen at 24–26 weeks gestation. This is performed by giving a small glucose load (50 g) and measuring serum glucose 1 h afterwards. If the screen is positive, a formal glucose tolerance test (3 h with a 75 or 100 g glucose load) is then done. "Pure" GDM usually resolves immediately after delivery; the women should be re-tested 6 weeks after delivery to make sure that it has resolved. These persons do have a strong likelihood (approaching 50%) of developing type 2 diabetes later in life, however.

Good control of diabetes during pregnancy is essential (whether preexisting or gestational). Fetuses of mothers with preexisting diabetes may develop organ malformations (e.g., neural tube and cardiac deformities) if control in the first trimester is poor. This problem does not occur in those with GDM because the organs are already formed by the time the glucose intolerance presents (late second trimester). Fetuses of mothers with both types of diabetes may develop macrosomia (a term meaning large babies). Larger is not necessarily better, especially in this case; macrosomia may result in delivery problems due to the neonates' large size.

It is strongly recommended that patients with preexisting diabetes have excellent control before considering pregnancy. Adequate contraceptive measures are necessary in those without optimal control; this cannot be emphasized enough. Success rates in pregnant patients with diabetes parallels that of the normal population when good control is present.

Many patients with GDM can be managed with diet alone. The dietary restriction is moderate and not enough to cause harm to the growing fetus. Insulin is necessary in patients with GDM who cannot achieve control with diet, and those with preexisting diabetes. Oral agents and other non-insulin therapies (e.g., metformin) have been used by some practitioners in pregnant patients with type 2 diabetes, but are not FDA approved for that purpose.

Monitoring diabetes

Diabetes management is more advanced today than ever before. Much of the improvement of care is due to the invention of small, portable glucose meters. These are small, battery-powered devices that allow the user to check his or her blood glucose. This is done by applying a small drop of capillary blood (from pricking the fingertip) to a disposable strip then inserted into the meter. This gives the user a way to monitor his or her readings and adjust treatment as necessary. Some meters contain a computer chip that allows downloading of the readings into a computer for detailed analysis. Also, some third-party payers (e.g., Medicare) require that the patient submit blood glucose logs (since they are paying for the test strips), and computer-generated records and the Internet facilitate this process.

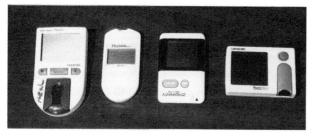

Home Blood Glucose Monitors

In the past, persons with diabetes monitored urine glucose. The first urine tests were complex proceedings that required boiling urine mixed with copper sulfate solution, which turned from blue to orange if glucose was present. Later, urine test strips became available. Urine glucose testing is not recommended today because of its inaccuracy, as the renal threshold for glucose varies among individuals.

Treatment goals depend on the individual. It would be ideal to keep all patients within the normal range all the time, but this is not possible in most people. One reason is that many treatments for diabetes (such as insulin) can cause hypoglycemia. The tighter the control, the more likely such reactions are. While a young, healthy adult might tolerate hypoglycemia well, an older individual might fall down and break his leg or have a motor vehicle

accident, for instance. Even in pediatric patients, this can be detrimental; excessive hypoglycemia in diabetic children has been linked to lower IQ.

A good rule of thumb is that the best degree of control without unacceptable hypoglycemia should be attained. Some will decide that they desire good diabetes control. Others, unfortunately, may not care much about their diabetes control and only wish to stay out of the hospital. Those with poor control are much more likely to develop complications than those with better control.

One simplistic way of describing levels of diabetes control to a patient is to make the analogy of traveling to the appliance store to buy a washer and dryer. You can purchase the cheap version, which may work well for a few years, but then break down. Or, you can buy the mid-priced version, which will last for perhaps 10 years. The top-of-the line model is the most expensive, but may last for a lifetime without breaking down. Diabetes control is the same way. Some of it boils down to luck. The cheap washer might last 25 years, but it probably would not. In the same line of thought, there are some patients with long histories of poorly controlled diabetes who have relatively few or no complications at all.

Overall, however, the odds clearly favor the person with well-controlled diabetes. In the end, it is best to recommend the best possible degree of control the patient can be reasonably expected to achieve without excessive hypoglycemia. But remember that not everyone will choose the "high-priced" model and some will settle for just staying out of the hospital. Some may have occupations (e.g., truck driver, heavy equipment operator) that would prohibit frequent hypoglycemia. However, the cost of intensive therapy in the long run helps prevent expensive complications and therapies for such (hemodialysis, foot surgeries, rehabilitation after stroke and amputation, hospitalizations, photocoagulation, etc.).

As mentioned, home blood glucose readings are essential data for individuals with diabetes. On the other hand, one can only check so many times per day. It is possible that the person is high or low during times that were not checked. Therefore, it is useful to have a secondary, backup test used to correlate with the other tests. Fortunately, such a test exists and is called glycated hemoglobin (HbA$_{1c}$). This test measures the amount of hemoglobin (the protein that carries oxygen through the blood) that glucose attaches to, and is reported as a percentage of the total hemoglobin. It is a useful index of long-term diabetic control and accurately reflects blood glucose values for the last 6 weeks. It is also now accepted as a diagnostic criterion for diabetes (a value ≥6.5% is diagnostic for diabetes).

It is good news if the patient's HbA$_{1c}$ level correlates with the average of his or her blood glucose readings. If the HbA$_{1c}$ is much higher than the glucose readings indicate, the patient may be experiencing hyperglycemia at times not checked. If it is much lower than the glucose meter readings, he or she may be having frequent hypoglycemia. Or, the meter may not be working properly, or the patient may be lying about his or her readings (this is common!). Rarely, a patient may have abnormal hemoglobin molecules that do not allow an accurate reading (e.g., sickle cell anemia, thalassemia). A relatively common condition that falsely elevates levels is iron deficiency anemia; the exact mechanism is unknown.

How do we know that good diabetes control matters? Well, for years, we did not; we really just hoped we were doing the right thing. Finally, in 1993, a study called the Diabetes Control and Complications Trial (DCCT) was completed. (I discuss this trial briefly in the section on evidence-based medicine.) This study took many years to complete and studied 1,500 patients with type 1 diabetes. Patients were randomized to receive either standard therapy (one or two injections per day—the midrange model (using our appliance analogy)) or intensive therapy (multiple daily injections or insulin infusion pump—the deluxe model). It was shown that intensively treated patients had a lower incidence of many complications. The United Kingdom Prospective Diabetes Study (UKPDS) was the first study demonstrating similar findings in patients with type 2 diabetes. Recent studies such as the Action to Control Cardiovascular Disease in Diabetes (ACCORD) trial showed that intensive glycemic control and intensive combination treatment of dyslipidemia reduced the rate of progression of diabetic retinopathy in patients with type 2 diabetes.

Excessively "tight" control may not always be advised, however. The ACCORD trial addressed the question if intensive control benefited patients with type 2 DM. The target "intensive" hemoglobin A$_{1c}$ was <6%, and the study showed that intensive control at this level actually *increased* total mortality (from hypoglycemia), so control at this level does not seem to be prudent for all. Studies showing aggressive inpatient control of diabetes initially aimed for a target of 110 mg/dL (6.05 mmol/L) or less; these studies revealed similar findings to ACCORD (that this level of control may result in adverse outcomes). Currently, the target of 140–180 mg/dL (7.7–9.9 mmol/L) for inpatient diabetes control is recommended (AACE–ADA Consensus Statement), with 110–140 mg/dL (6.05–7.7 mmol/L) being acceptable for some patients.

Overly aggressive control of diabetes may have unwanted consequences in other populations as well. Some studies have shown decreased IQ in children intensively treated for diabetes; the drop in IQ is presumably due to more frequent hypoglycemic episodes.

Complications of diabetes

Before effective treatments for diabetes were available, most patients died before they could develop complications (most of which were unknown because patients did not live very long anyway). Even after insulin was discovered in 1921, it was many years before common complications were discovered. The initial exuberance over effective treatment of diabetes was later tempered by the recognition that such complications developed in patients with poor control. These were much more frequent in the early years of insulin therapy because blood glucose monitoring was not available.

Patients with diabetes are more prone to certain medical problems than those without the disorder. These can be divided into two broad categories: microvascular (small vessel) and macrovascular (large vessel) disease. Microvascular diseases include diabetic retinopathy (eye disease), nephropathy (kidney disease), and neuropathy (nerve disease). Macrovascular disease includes coronary artery disease (angina pectoris and myocardial infarction), cerebrovascular disease (stroke), and peripheral vascular disease.

What causes the complications of diabetes? Although extremely high glucose levels may cause ketoacidosis and even death in severe circumstances, glucose itself does not appear to be the cause of chronic complications. The pathogenesis of diabetic complications remains poorly understood. Evidence indicates that many diabetic complications may be caused by advanced glycation endproducts (AGEs). Long-term hyperglycemia causes glycation of many proteins. These products themselves may cause protein damage dysfunction, or may cause production of deleterious products, such as tumor necrosis factor and interleukins.

Diabetic neuropathy

Neuropathy is a common complication of diabetes that can result in significant morbidity. It is divided into peripheral nerve (somatic) neuropathies and autonomic (central nervous system) neuropathies. The most common form of neuropathy is a distal sensory neuropathy that results in distal numbness ("stocking" distribution). Pain may also occur with this type of neuropathy, and it may be resistant to treatment. A less common form of neuropathy is a proximal motor and sensory neuropathy (amyotrophy). A common form of autonomic neuropathy is hypoglycemia unawareness, in which the patient is unaware that his or her glucose is low. This may have devastating consequences, as the person may suffer a seizure, wreck a motor vehicle, or even die without intervention by another person. Sometimes autonomic neuropathies keep the patient's heart rate from increasing in response to exercise (fixed heart rate). Diabetic gastroparesis is another form of diabetic autonomic neuropathy that causes delayed gastric emptying. Because stomach contents are not readily emptied, nausea, vomiting, and early satiety (feeling full before the entire meal is eaten) may occur. Since food is absorbed erratically, poor diabetes control often develops. Medications (prokinetics) such as metoclopramide and erythromycin are available that can help this problem, but results with medication are often unsatisfactory. Gastric pacing (a procedure where a "pacemaker" (similar to a cardiac pacemaker) supplies electrical stimulation to the stomach (replacing lost nerve signals)) has shown efficacy in some patients.

The best treatment of diabetic neuropathy is improvement of glycemic control. Tricyclic antidepressants such as amitriptyline and anticonvulsants such as gabapentin and carbamazepine may be useful. Narcotic analgesics should be avoided, as they are not very effective for this type of pain and can be addicting.

The diabetic foot

Patients with diabetes, neuropathy, and peripheral vascular disease are much more likely to develop foot problems. A small abrasion or penetrating wound, while only a nuisance to normal persons, can be devastating to those with diabetes with these complications. An infected foot ulcer, for instance, can lead to weeks of hospitalization for antibiotic therapy or even amputation.

The health care provider should always look at the patient's feet during the examination. This often uncovers problems such as calluses or small ulcerations that were not previously known to the patient. Appropriate measures (e.g., antibiotics, referral to a podiatrist or pedorthist) are then possible before the problems become severe.

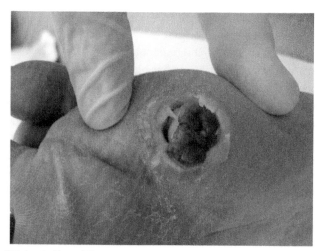

Diabetic Foot Ulcer

Diabetic retinopathy

Probably the most feared complication of diabetes is blindness. Millions of patients go blind each year as a result of this disease. With optimal control, however, the incidence of retinopathy decreases, and effective treatment is available.

There are two basic types of retinopathy: nonproliferative and proliferative. Nonproliferative or "background" retinopathy is seen in many patients after many years with diabetes. It does not cause vision loss, and if it does not progress, is of minimal significance in the peripheral visual field. It may cause problems in the central visual field (fovea) if macular edema (swelling in the foveal area) occurs.

Proliferative retinopathy is much more ominous. This leads to neovascularization (new blood vessel growth) and possible vitreous hemorrhage (bleeding into the eye) and retinal detachment. This may lead to vision loss and blindness. Fortunately, this can sometimes be prevented by laser photocoagulation (destroying new blood vessels in the peripheral field). This does not affect central vision. Peripheral and night vision may be slightly diminished by repeated laser treatments. Intraocular instillation of novel anti-vascular endothelial growth factors (anti-VEGFs) such as bevacizumab have shown promise in ameliorating progressive retinopathy.

All patients with diabetes must see a qualified optometrist or ophthalmologist on a regular basis (at least annually for a dilated eye exam) to detect any new problems, as often they do not present to the patient until disaster strikes (e.g., retinal hemorrhage with retinal detachment and vision loss).

Diabetic nephropathy

Diabetic nephropathy is another small vessel or microvascular disease, like retinopathy. Patients with diabetes for many years may begin to suffer early kidney damage. The first stage is manifested by hyperfiltration (increased filtration through the kidney). This is measured by performing a 24-h urine collection for creatinine and measuring the creatinine clearance, which is a rough estimate of glomerular filtration rate (GFR). The normal value is between 70 and 120 mL/min. A patient with stage I nephropathy might have a creatinine clearance of, say, 180 mL/min. The initial response to your patient might be, "Fantastic! Your kidney function is 150% of normal! You have kidney function to spare!" This is, however, not fantastic at all; it is in reality a sinister harbinger of possible worsening kidney disease. The kidney may also leak small amounts of protein, or microalbumin, at this point. Fortunately, the nephropathy is potentially reversible at this time with certain measures. Certain types of blood pressure medications, angiotensin converting-enzyme inhibitors (ACEI), and angiotensin receptor blockers (ARBs), help reverse nephropathy at this stage, even if the blood pressure is normal. As nephropathy progresses, microalbuminuria (small amounts of protein, <500 mg/day) persist. In the next stage, protein persists at over 500 mg/day (overt proteinuria), GFR decreases (meaning decreased kidney function), and hypertension occurs. At this stage, the kidney damage is clearly irreversible, and all patients will progress to complete kidney failure in time. Even at this late stage, however, the progression to complete failure can be slowed by good blood pressure and glucose control, and restriction of protein in the diet.

Those with end-stage nephropathy have complete kidney failure and will die without treatment. Available treatments include renal replacement therapy (dialysis) or kidney transplantation. Billions of dollars are spent yearly on dialysis treatments for diabetic patients, making this the most expensive diabetic complication to treat. One type of dialysis is called hemodialysis, in which the patient is connected to a dialysis machine by an arteriovenous fistula in the arm for several hours three times weekly. Another type is called continuous ambulatory peritoneal dialysis (CAPD). This works by using the peritoneal membrane of the abdomen as a filter. A catheter is placed permanently in the abdomen, and large amounts of peritoneal dialysis fluid are infused into this space. This process is much slower than hemodialysis because it works by passive diffusion. The large peritoneal dialysis bags are also quite cumbersome, but this procedure has the advantage of performing it at home. Some patients prefer this to hemodialysis. One problem with CAPD is that the dialysate (fluid) bags contain large amounts of glucose, which may interfere with diabetes control. Sometimes, insulin is placed in the CAPD bags, which may help control. However, the introduction of needles into the CAPD bags (a sterile solution) increases the likelihood of infection.

Life expectancy in patients with diabetes on dialysis is extremely poor, with the mean survival after beginning therapy being less than 2 years. It appears that patients with diabetes on dialysis have such severe vascular disease elsewhere that life expectancy is dismal; good control of glucose and hypertension may help prolong survival.

Renal transplants are preferred in patients who are good candidates. Poor candidates include those who have severe cardiovascular disease and are morbidly obese (they might not tolerate surgery very well). The best transplants occur with a kidney from a related donor (e.g., a sibling). Living donors in good health may safely donate one kidney, as the remaining kidney is sufficient for them. Cadaveric (from a deceased donor) transplants are generally less successful than those from relatives. Patients undergoing transplantation need powerful anti-rejection drugs the rest of their lives. Those with successful transplants no longer require dialysis. However, the need for organs unfortunately far outweighs the supply currently available.

Diabetic ketoacidosis

Diabetic ketoacidosis (DKA) may occur in type 1 patients who are without insulin for long periods of time. In the normal person, basal insulin levels allow balanced glucose homeostasis. With lack of insulin, the body thinks it is in a starved state since glucose cannot get into the cells (when in fact the concentration in the blood is quite high). As a result, the body starts breaking down fats and proteins, producing waste products such as ketones in an effort to gain energy from these sources. This propagates a vicious cycle—the body has plenty of glucose in the blood, but cannot use it.

The breakdown products of these alternate energy sources (e.g., ketones) eventually results in ketoacidosis. Medium-chain ketones have a fruity odor, and the breath of these patients often smells fruity. The very high glucose concentration in the blood acts as an osmotic diuretic and causes massive fluid losses from the body via the urine. These patients are therefore very dehydrated in addition to being acidotic. Death results if untreated; this is how patients died before the discovery of insulin in 1921. (They did not live long enough to develop the common complications we see today.)

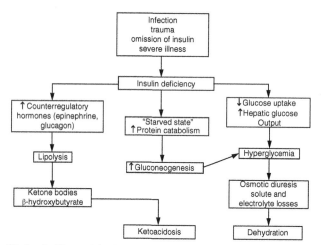

Diabetic Ketoacidosis

One of the most common reasons for ketoacidosis is infection (e.g., pneumonia, urinary tract infection). Another common cause is omission of insulin on sick days. Patients sometimes think that if they are sick and not eating, they should omit their insulin. Nothing is further from the truth! Even persons not eating need some insulin to maintain normal bodily functions. The ill person should instead follow sick day rules that involve taking the scheduled insulin plus supplemental soluble insulin every few hours if high.

DKA is treated with fluids and insulin. Large amounts of fluids (e.g., 5–10 L) may be necessary to restore the lost fluids (i.e., with 0.9% normal saline). Older patients with diminished cardiac reserve may need special monitoring to prevent congestive heart failure and pulmonary edema.

Insulin is most commonly administered as an intravenous infusion for DKA, and is continued until the acidosis resolves. Subcutaneous insulin must be started at least an hour before the intravenous insulin is discontinued, due to the latter's short half-life (under 10 min).

Hyperosmolar nonketotic syndrome (HNKS)

Hyperosmolar nonketotic syndrome (HNKS) is another syndrome of acute metabolic decompensation in patients with diabetes. Like those with DKA, these patients have severe hyperglycemia (often >1,000 mg/dL) and dehydration; unlike DKA, ketoacidosis is absent.

HNKS is commonly the presenting manifestation of diabetes in elderly patients and is typically associated with a concurrent illness (e.g., infection, myocardial infarction, stroke).

HNKS differs from DKA since patients with the former have sufficient insulin to prevent lipolysis and metabolic acidosis. However, there is enough relative insulin deficiency to cause hyperglycemia and protein/carbohydrate catabolism, leading to osmotic diuresis with fluid and electrolyte depletion.

The treatment of HNKS includes fluid and electrolyte repletion. Intravenous insulin is also necessary in most patients. Subcutaneous insulin is started after the acute metabolic decompensation resolves, and underlying conditions such as infection are treated.

Therapy of type 1 diabetes

Patients with type 1 diabetes had a dismal future before the discovery of insulin. All patients died, but life could be (miserably) prolonged by a year or two by administering starvation diets that deprived the patient of glucose. It was discovered in 1889 that total pancreatectomy produced diabetes in dogs, and the concept of a glucose-lowering substance located in the pancreatic islets of Langerhans was postulated. After many years of fruitless investigation, insulin was discovered in 1921 at the University of Toronto by Fred Banting (a surgeon); Charles Best (a medical student); James Collip (a biochemist); and J.J.R. Macleod (a physiologist). Banting and Macleod received the Nobel Prize for their efforts. Their insulin was soluble or regular insulin (pure human insulin without any additives). When injected as a subcutaneous depot, its onset of action was 0.5–2 h, with a peak in 3–4 h and duration of 6–8 h; it was therefore termed short-acting or rapid-acting insulin. While life saving to millions of diabetics, the "regular" insulin's short duration of action was inconvenient.

It was then discovered that the addition of certain impurities to regular insulin resulted in delayed absorption. This gave birth to the intermediate- and long-acting series of insulins. One retarding agent was zinc, used in the now-discontinued Lente series (Lente, Ultralente, Semilente). Another is the protein protamine, used in NPH (also called N) insulin, which is still available.

A different approach was then taken once insulin could be synthesized and modified; instead of retarding insulin absorption with impurities, scientists engineered synthetic long-acting insulins (which are absorbed much more slowly than rapid-acting insulins). Currently available long-acting analogs include insulins detemir and glargine. While their pharmacokinetics in theory are superior to NPH (the only currently available intermediate-acting human insulin), they are much more expensive to produce and, for some patients, do not produce superior results. One disadvantage of the long-acting analogs is that, unlike NPH, they cannot be mixed with short-acting insulin, often leading to additional injections per day; however, most patients feel that the superiority of these insulins outweighs that disadvantage (insulin syringes are very fine and short these days).

Insulin is a large peptide hormone that is unfortunately rapidly degraded in the gastrointestinal tract, making oral administration difficult. At this time it must be given subcutaneously (under the skin). Depending on the preparation, subcutaneous absorption may take place within minutes or within hours. Some preparations (like insulin detemir and glargine) last almost an entire day. Intravenous insulin administration is impractical for non-hospitalized patients, as the short half-life of insulin in serum (about seven minutes) requires a continuous infusion for efficacy.

Insulin is also well absorbed through the peritoneal cavity and may be administered this way in certain patients (e.g., those on dialysis). Other methods of insulin administration (e.g., inhaled aerosol) are being studied experimentally. An inhalable insulin was briefly available from 2006 to 2007, but was removed from the market for numerous reasons, among them poor sales and a cumbersome, complex delivery system. Another inhaled insulin preparation was approved by the FDA in 2014.

In the last decade, scientists have sought more rapid-acting insulins that could more closely parallel native insulin secretion. Regular (R) insulin sometimes lasts for 4–6 h, producing unpredictable hypoglycemia in certain patients. By synthetically modifying human insulin, rapid insulin analogs were created in the early 1990s. The first such marketed insulin, lispro, takes action in only 15 min and peaks in 30 min to 1 h. These insulins are advantageous, since they may be taken right before a meal (vs 30 min for R insulin). Other synthetic insulins, aspart and glulisine, have similar properties. Like detemir and glargine, they are synthetic analogs, but with very rapid onset of action. The reason for this is that regular insulin aggregates into a hexameric state in the vial or pen at the solution's concentration; yet, it only can be absorbed in the monomeric state, and must reach a certain concentration before dissociating into monomers. The rapid-acting analogs aggregate less avidly, meaning that they dissociate into monomers at higher concentrations and are absorbed more rapidly.

Insulin Pharmacokinetics

Insulin	Onset	Peak Activity	Duration of Action (h)
NPH[a]	2–4 h	4–9 h	10–16
Glargine	2–4 h	Minimal	20–24
Detemir	2–4 h	8–10 h	16–20
Regular[a] (U-100)	30–60 min	2–3 h	5–8
Regular[a] (U-500)	30–60 min	4–8 h	12–14
Lispro, aspart, glulisine	5–15 min	30–90 min	4–6

[a]Human insulin.

For many decades, insulin was produced from beef and hog pancreases. Although these proteins differ slightly from human insulin, they work well in humans. Since they are foreign proteins, however, a small percentage of people developed allergic reactions to animal insulins. Another concern was that the supply of animal pancreases might someday be exhausted, leading to inadequate insulin supplies. For these reasons, all insulin available today is synthetic human insulin of recombinant DNA origin. It is made by inserting the gene for human insulin into bacteria or yeast, which then manufactures the insulin.

U-500 regular insulin (500 units/mL; other insulins are U-100, or 100 units/mL) is a special formulation of concentrated insulin used in highly insulin-resistant patients. Its unique absorption gives it properties of both a short- and an intermediate-acting insulin. Due to its high concentration, it is for "special use" only as it can be hazardous if not drawn up and injected properly. It is useful in patients in whom injecting very large amounts of insulin is either impractical or not efficacious.

Diet therapy

Good nutrition is as important as medication for good control of diabetes. In those with type 2 diabetes, it is the preferred initial therapy (those with type 1 also need insulin, obviously, but good nutrition is important here as well). Unfortunately, many patients who are willing to take insulin or non-insulin agents are unable or unwilling to follow a proper diet. The most feared professional in the diabetes clinic is often not the physician, but the officious dietitian, who asks patients to make undesired dietary modifications. Fortunately, diet prescriptions (yes, food is like a drug to a person with diabetes) are more flexible today than ever before. In the past, they were very rigid and required patients to weigh food. Now they center on total amounts of calories and food groups. The diet should be tailored to the patient—some may be unable to follow an excessively complex diet plan.

The simplest way of following a sensible diet is the food pyramid. Foods at the top of the pyramid should be eaten sparingly or not at all (high fat foods, desserts, alcoholic beverages). Those at the bottom (e.g., cereals) can be eaten in much larger portions. This is a relatively simple plan that most people can follow.

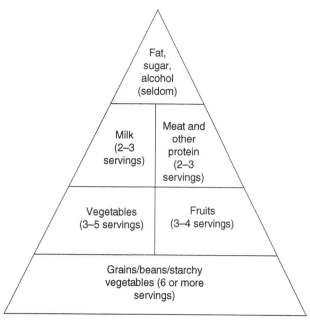

The Food Pyramid

An exchange list diet is a method where foods are grouped into carbohydrate, meat/meat substitute, and fat groups. Exchange lists are a simple way of making food choices. Each person can eat a certain number from each exchange for each meal. For example, if another carbohydrate is desired, the person simply makes a substitution for the equivalent amount of another exchange.

Patients with type 2 diabetes are often overweight and the goal is a modest weight loss.

Weight loss of 1–2 lb/week is desired.

Insulin pumps

Many patients with diabetes use insulin pumps. These devices supply insulin via continuous subcutaneous insulin infusion (CSII), a method by which short-acting insulin is continuously infused by the pump. Pumps are small, beeper-sized devices that contain insulin, and deliver it to the patient through a thin plastic tube inserted under the skin at the one end. An implantable pump has been studied experimentally. This is implanted inside the body, like a pacemaker, and is refilled periodically with insulin delivered through a subcutaneous infusion port. This is programmed with an external device much in the same way as an external pump, and the insulin is released into the peritoneal cavity (where it is absorbed almost as rapidly as intravenous insulin). These are not currently available for commercial use and are currently only used in research trials.

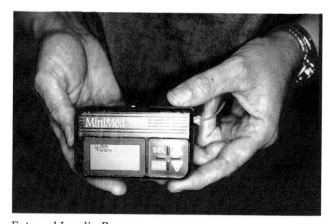

External Insulin Pump

The patient programs the external pump to give a set amount of basal insulin, and gives additional insulin (boluses) before meals. The advantage of the pump is that very small amounts of insulin can be given accurately (in increments of 0.05 units). With conventional syringes, insulin can be given only in 1-unit increments. A set meal bolus (e.g., 2 units) may be given, or may be given in an increment depending on a set amount of carbohydrate; for example, a patient might be given 1 unit of insulin for each 10 g of carbohydrate. "Carb counting" in this manner obviously requires that the patient know how much carbohydrate is on the plate before programming the amount. Yet, this form of administering a meal bolus allows the greatest flexibility in the regimen. (Carb counting can be used for standard insulin injections, but does not allow as much "exact" titration given the inherent limitations in administering very small amounts of insulin with a syringe and needle.)

Some patients and providers have misconceptions about pumps. A commonly held notion is that the pump gives insulin by itself without intervention by the wearer. The basal rate function does give insulin continuously, but the user has to set it. And meal boluses are not given without user instruction. The pump has no way of knowing what the wearer's glucose is (unless a continuous sensor is used; more on this later), and so this must be checked in the same way as always (with a glucose meter); there are meters that wirelessly link to the pump, but this method still requires effort. Pump therapy is actually much more complicated and expensive than conventional injections. In return, however, it allows more flexibility for the motivated user.

Using an insulin pump is like comparing a Chevrolet sedan to an Indianapolis 500 race car. Conventional insulin injections are to some extent like the Chevy: almost anybody can drive it acceptably under typical conditions. But this vehicle, while providing basic transportation, lacks the flexibility to deal with unusual situations (that some persons will not face anyway). The IndyCar, on the other hand, can go over 200 mile/h and is a much more sophisticated machine. Without adequate training, however, the average person driving it is likely to have a wreck or other undesirable outcome. The same is true with a pump—those poorly suited for a pump are likely to have more problems than they did using injections. Candidates for insulin pumps should be selected carefully: they are not for everyone. They are a poor choice for someone who is not willing to put proper time and effort into it.

Pumps are generally used in patients with type 1 diabetes, although some patients with type 2 may also benefit. Current pumps are unable to deliver the large amounts of insulin necessary for very insulin-resistant individuals; insulin U-500 has been used in selected insulin-resistant patients with good results. Also, patients with type 2 diabetes may also be less prone to hypoglycemia and therefore do not often require the benefits of the pump.

Continuous glucose monitoring (CGM) via an attached sensor has increased the toolkit available for practitioners to more closely monitor diabetes. The continuous glucose sensor has been available as an adjunct to self-glucose monitoring for many years. While a majority of patients using continuous glucose sensor (CGS) are on insulin pumps, this is not a requirement. The CGS sensor is inserted into subcutaneous tissue and measures glucose in interstitial fluid, giving near-real time (interstitial fluid glucose lags behind blood glucose by about 15 min) readings to help troubleshoot difficult problems. It is a useful adjunct to therapy in selected patients.

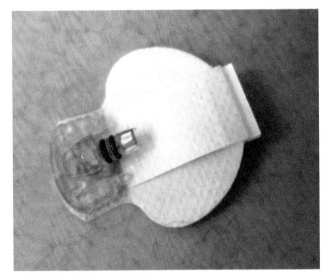

Continuous Insulin Sensor

Team approach to diabetes

Good diabetes treatment usually requires more than what the physician can provide. Unlike many other medical disorders, the patient has to do most of the work; it is not as simple as taking a pill or injection. This complex regimen requires that patients be well educated about their illness. The diabetes team may consist of the following: Physician; diabetes educator; nurse practitioner; registered dietitian; podiatrist; ophthalmologist/optometrist; vascular surgeon; nephrologist; social worker; pharmacist; and mental health/counseling services.

A certified diabetes educator (CDE) should be the primary educational resource in teaching patients about diabetes care. These are health care professionals (physicians, registered nurses, dietitians, or pharmacists) who have an interest, and have received advanced training, in the care and education of patients with diabetes. They must take a rigorous qualifying examination and be periodically recertified.

Non-insulin agents for diabetes

In addition to insulin, there are many other agents useful in the treatment of diabetes. These are often called oral hypoglycemic agents or antihyperglycemic agents, although the glucagon-like peptide-1 (GLP-1) agonists and pramlintide are given subcutaneously. The non-insulin agents can be divided into several classes.

Sulfonylureas were first discovered in the 1940s during World War II when new antibiotics were being developed. Researchers found that several patients receiving these experimental antibiotics (chemically similar to sulfonamide antibiotics) suffered hypoglycemia. Carbutamide was the first sulfonylurea used, but had adverse clinical effects. The so-called first-generation agents were introduced in the late 1950s and included tolbutamide and chlorpropamide. Acetohexamide and tolazamide were introduced later. The second-generation sulfonylureas were then introduced; these include glyburide and glipizide; the newest second-generation agent is glimepiride.

Sulfonylureas act by sensitizing the pancreatic β cells to glucose, which results in increased insulin secretion. Intact β cells are obviously required, and so they are not useful in patients with type 1 diabetes (who completely lack exogenous insulin).

Glyburide, A Sulfonylurea

Since sulfonylureas fall into the category of insulin secretagogues, hypoglycemia may occur, especially in the elderly; this is one reason these drugs are no longer considered first-line agents, despite their efficacy. Patients with prolonged hypoglycemia require admission to the hospital due to the relatively long duration of action of sulfonylureas. Chlorpropamide, specifically, has a very long half-life and generally should not be used. Because of these problems, sulfonylureas are often not used as first-line therapies for type 2 diabetes any longer and have been removed from many hospital inpatient formularies. One advantage is their low cost, since they have been available for decades. Long-acting preparations (once daily) are available.

Another class of drugs, the meglitinides ("glinides"), are benzoic acid derivatives that include repaglinide and nateglinide. Although structurally different than sulfonylureas, they are also insulin secretagogues and may be thought of as "fast-acting sulfonylureas." They are generally taken before meals. Because they increase insulin secretion (like sulfonylureas), they may also induce hypoglycemia. Meglitinides may be combined with other oral agents or insulin.

Nateglinide, A Meglitinide

Biguanides are a class of drugs that increase insulin sensitivity and decrease hepatic glucose output. Metformin is a biguanide and a very useful drug for the treatment of type 2 diabetes. It is derived from a compound found in the plant *Galega officinalis* (French lilac), which has been used since the Middle Ages for relieving symptoms of type 2 diabetes. Metformin may be used by itself or in combination with other oral agents or insulin. Because it does not increase insulin secretion, it does not cause hypoglycemia. Like other non-secretagogue agents, it may increase the effectiveness of other agents (such as insulin and sulfonylureas), and may, therefore, potentiate the hypoglycemic effects of these drugs; doses of other drugs may need to be decreased when starting metformin. Its most common adverse side effect is gastrointestinal: it occasionally causes mild diarrhea and increased flatulence. Only rarely, however, is this severe enough to necessitate discontinuation of the drug.

Metformin, A Biguanide

The most serious side effect of metformin therapy is lactic acidosis, which is, fortunately, quite rare. Metformin increases the body's lactic acid production to a slight extent, which is of no significant consequence in normal persons. However, in those with significant kidney or liver disease, this complication can rarely occur, and may result in death. This drug therefore should not be used in such patients and in those with marginal renal function who may suffer a transient decline in renal function (e.g., patients receiving iodinated contrast dyes for radiologic or cardiovascular procedures). It is a very safe drug in normal patients without these problems.

A novel class of drugs includes the thiazolidinediones (TZDs or glitazones). These drugs act by increasing the body's sensitivity to insulin by acting on adipose, muscle, and liver cells to enhance glucose utilization, thus attacking the fundamental problem in patients with type 2 diabetes. The mechanism by which they work is not fully understood, but they seem to activate one or more peroxisome proliferator-activated receptors (PPARs), which regulate gene expression. The drugs currently available are pioglitazone and rosiglitazone. Troglitazone, the first marketed drug, was associated with hepatic disease in rare cases and was taken off the market in the United States in early 2000. Rosiglitazone has been associated with adverse cardiovascular outcomes by some studies. Because of the experience with troglitazone, however, routine serum liver enzyme studies are recommended in patients taking current TZD drugs.

Incretin mimetics or GLP-1 agonists (exenatide and liraglutide) are administered subcutaneously. They were first identified as a substance (exendin-4) isolated from the saliva of the venomous lizard *Heloderma suspectum* (Gila monster) found in the southwestern United States. GLP-1 receptor agonists increase glucose-stimulated insulin secretion, suppress glucagon, and slow gastric emptying. However, unlike other agents that increase insulin secretion, GLP-1 agonists do not cause weight gain, and most patients experience some weight loss and appetite suppression. They also do not cause hypoglycemia. They are approved for the treatment of type 2 diabetes in patients not sufficiently controlled with diet, exercise, or oral agents. Exenatide requires two daily injections while liraglutide requires one (there is now an extended-release preparation of exenatide that can be given once weekly). They are not generally used as monotherapy and are contraindicated in renal failure. Because they delay gastric emptying, they may slow the oral absorption of other drugs and may cause nausea and vomiting in some patients.

Sitagliptin, linagliptin, saxagliptin, and alogliptin are dipeptidyl peptidase-4 (DPP-IV) inhibitors that are approved as initial pharmacologic therapy for the treatment of type 2 diabetes. They decrease the degradation of GLP-1 and promote its endogenous effect, so they act in a similar manner to GLP-1 agonists. However, because of modest glucose lowering effectiveness and high cost, they are more typically used as a second agent in those who do not respond to a single agent, such as a sulfonylurea, metformin or aTZD; or as a third agent when dual therapy with metformin and a sulfonylurea does not provide adequate glycemic control. Linagliptin and saxagliptin have the advantage that they are not cleared renally and can be used by patients with chronic

kidney disease (CKD). Like GLP-1 agonists, they cause insulin secretion without hypoglycemia or weight gain. Since they have a similar mechanism of action to GLP-1 agonists, the two are not used together.

Sitagliptin, A DPP-IV Inhibitor

A protein called amylin (human islet amyloid polypeptide, IAPP), is secreted by the β cells and its secretion is lost in type 1 diabetes; this compound was felt to be unimportant for decades but there has been renewed interest in the unique properties of this protein. Pramlintide, a synthetic analogue of human islet amyloid polypeptide, lowers postprandial glucose levels when used with insulin, and can be used in combination with insulin for patients with both type 1 and type 2 diabetes. Pramlintide delays gastric emptying, increases satiety, reduces food intake, and decreases postprandial glucagon secretion; unlike the GLP-1 agonists, it does not alter insulin levels. In trials of patients with type 1 diabetes, the addition of pramlintide to insulin therapy decreased postprandial glucose, hemoglobin A_{1c}, insulin use, and weight. Like the GLP-1 agonists, pramlintide delays gastric emptying and can delay absorption of oral medications. But it remains the only non-insulin agent which is a useful adjunct to insulin therapy in type 1 diabetics.

The α-glucosidase inhibitors are another class of non-insulin agents. These drugs (acarbose and miglitol) inhibit α-glucosidase, an enzyme found in the brush border of the small intestine. These drugs inhibit the cleavage of oligosaccharides (such as sucrose) into simple sugars. This effectively leads to decreased absorption of these sugars after a meal. Glucose absorption is not affected; patients must treat hypoglycemia with glucose, and not sucrose (found in most sugared drinks and candy) or other more complex sugars, as they will be ineffective. A frequent side effect of acarbose or miglitol therapy is increased flatulence, due to colonic bacterial digestion of the unabsorbed oligosaccharides. They are useful in selected type 2 diabetics with elevated postprandial glucose levels.

Canagliflozin and dapagliflozin are novel inhibitors of SGLT2 (subtype 2 sodium-glucose transport protein), which is responsible for at least 90% of the glucose reabsorption in the kidney. Blocking this transporter causes blood glucose to be eliminated through the urine and decreases serum glucose levels. Interestingly, they appear to have an effect on lowering systolic blood pressure, given their ability to cause osmotic diuresis.

While typically used to treat lipids, bile acid sequestrants (such as colesevelam) have a very modest glucose-lowering effect. The dopamine agonist bromocriptine also has minimal glucose-lowering properties (less than 0.5% reduction in hemoglobin A_{1c}), so it is not commonly used for this purpose. It might be useful in patients requiring bromocriptine for another purpose (e.g., prolactinoma).

Average Reduction in Hemoglobin A_{1c} for Non-insulin Diabetes Therapies

Metformin	1.5%
Insulin secretagogues (sulfonlyureas, meglitinides)	1.5–2.0%
Incretin mimetics (GLP-1 agonists—exenatide, liraglutide)	1.0–1.5%
DPP-IV inhibitors (sitagliptin, linagliptin, saxagliptin alogliptin)	0.6–1.0%
α-Glucosidase inhibitors (acarbose, miglitol)	1.0%
Amylin agonists (pramlintide)	0.5–1.0%
TZDs (pioglitazone, rosiglitazone)	1.0–1.4%
Bile acid sequestrants (colesevelam, colestipol)	<0.5%
SGLT2 inhibitors (canagliflozin, dapagliflozin)	0.5–1.2%
Dopamine agonist (bromocriptine)	0.5%

Curing and preventing diabetes

Diabetes is a tremendous medical and economic burden on the patient and society. It is a ubiquitous endocrine disorder that seriously impacts health and reduces life span and quality of life; an estimated 16 million Americans (and 135 million people worldwide) currently have diabetes. The World Health Organization projects the latter will grow to 300 million people by the year 2025. Many more have impaired glucose tolerance or impaired fasting glucose and are at high risk for atherosclerotic disease and diabetes. Approximately one out of every seven health care dollars is spent on diabetes and its complications. Therefore, it should consequently be no surprise that there are many efforts underway to cure or prevent this disease.

From a theoretical perspective, type 1 diabetes seems the simplest to cure. We can manufacture synthetic human insulin and a variety of analogs with unique properties, so all that is necessary is to replace insulin in a physiologic manner. This is, of course, much easier said than done—current technologies only provide an approximation of what a normal person's body does.

Currently, the closest thing to a cure for type 1 diabetes is restoration of the patient's β cell mass by transplantation of the whole pancreas (pancreas transplantation) or of the islets themselves (islet cell transplantation). In whole pancreas transplantation, a cadaveric organ is used (a living donor is, obviously, impossible, as that person needs his or her pancreas). Islet cell transplantation is more difficult; this involves purification of the delicate islets from a donor and infusing them into the portal vein. These functional islets "set up shop" in the liver and begin sensing glucose levels and secreting insulin, just as if they were in the pancreas. The advantage of these procedures is the achievement of normal or near-normal glycemic control with freedom from insulin, thus reducing the likelihood of long-term complications and improving the quality of life.

Unfortunately, both the foreign pancreas and islet cells will be rejected by the recipient's immune system without potent immunosuppressive drugs. Because of the risks of these agents, pancreas and islet cell transplants were once reserved for patients who also required another organ (e.g., a kidney); because immunosuppressive drugs would be required anyway, transplantation carries little additional risk (beyond that of the surgical procedure itself). Nonetheless, several centers are now performing pancreas-only transplantation for those with severe diabetic complications. The 5-year survival of a whole pancreas transplant is about 60%, while islet cell graft longevity is lower. In any case, patients with a functional graft have a significantly better quality of life than before. A better understanding of ways to overcome immune rejection will lead to improved survival of these grafts. Even if the immune problems can be solved, there are far too few donor pancreases or pancreatic islets to meet the needs of the millions with type 1 diabetes. So other methods of procurement (e.g., stem cell research) must be found if a true cure is to be realized. Many researchers are devoting their careers to this aspect of endocrinology.

Another approach is to improve insulin pumps by creating truly "closed-loop" systems. Currently, the pumps require a great deal of intervention by the wearer (checking blood glucose, programming insulin boluses). It would be wonderful if an implantable insulin sensor was available that could provide feedback to the pump with fewer necessary interventions. At this time, sensors that survive in the body for long periods of time are not available, but are being studied experimentally; the currently available continuous glucose sensors are much improved from even 5 years ago, but still require relatively "high maintenance" and must be changed every few days.

Several clinical trials have also examined the prospects of preventing the development of type 1 diabetes. First-degree relatives of those with type 1 DM may enroll in these trials, and they are monitored for development of islet cell autoantibodies and/or hyperglycemia. Individuals who develop autoantibodies and hyperglycemia may receive an immunosuppressive drug, which appears to at least delay the onset of type 1 diabetes. Thus far, results of these trials have been very disappointing. The prospect of preventing type 2 diabetes (by identifying individuals at risk and intervening with lifestyle interventions) seems more promising.

HYPOGLYCEMIA

"Hypoglycemia" is often a disorder poorly understood by physicians and other health care providers, as well as patients. Many patients casually note during the medical history that they or another family member has "low blood sugar," and needs to keep something around to eat at all times. In reality, hypoglycemia is a rare disorder that most providers are unlikely to encounter, except in the instance of insulin- or sulfonylurea/meglitinide-treated diabetics. It is a commonly touted cause of societal ills in the lay press, and many sources in print and on the Internet exist to propagate the notion of this disorder.

When most people think of hypoglycemia, they think or postprandial or reactive hypoglycemia. The normal response to an oral glucose load is secretion of an appropriate amount of insulin by the pancreas, resulting in euglycemia. In those with true reactive hypoglycemia,

the insulin response is exaggerated, leading to postprandial hypoglycemia with resultant symptoms. True reactive hypoglycemia is quite rare, and often over-diagnosed, sometimes by misuse of the 100-g glucose tolerance test. Even if reactive hypoglycemia does exist, it is not a life-threatening disorder, and not a cause of constant fatigue and suffering, and may be managed with smaller, more frequent meals and avoidance of concentrated sweets.

Patients with abnormal gastric emptying (e.g., postgastrectomy) have rapid "dumping" of food into the intestinal tract, which may result in hyperinsulinism. They may in fact have severe postprandial hypoglycemia. Treatment involves smaller, more frequent meals; acarbose or miglitol (α-glucosidase inhibitors) can reduce carbohydrate absorption and may be helpful.

Another important note is that those persons with impaired glucose tolerance occasionally have delayed insulin release 1 or 2h after a meal, resulting in mild postprandial hypoglycemia. Treatment is weight loss and dietary management. It is common for a patient with type 2 diabetes to mention that he or she had "hypoglycemia" when younger.

A much more ominous form of hypoglycemia is fasting hypoglycemia, which occurs in the patient who has gone without food for several hours (although severe postprandial hypoglycemia can occur in patients with surgical alterations). Typically the patient feels worst in the morning and feels better after eating. This type of hypoglycemia is associated with either insulin hypersecretion or glucose underproduction.

An insulin-secreting islet cell tumor (insulinoma) is a rare cause of fasting hypoglycemia. These patients are prone to spontaneous attacks of weakness, hypoglycemic symptoms, and even syncope, seizures, and death if untreated. Treatment involves removal of the offending tumor. Other tumors can produce hypoglycemia by a humoral factor (such as insulin-like growth factor II (IGF-II)).

Another recognized type of hypoglycemia is called noninsulinoma pancreatogenous hypoglycemia syndrome (NIPHS). These patients often exhibit severe hypoglycemia after meals and demonstrate β cell hypertrophy. This syndrome can rarely occur after certain bariatric procedures and may require pancreatectomy if severe; since bariatric procedures have become more common, NIPHS is being seen more frequently. Again, α-glucosidase inhibitors can be useful.

Another important cause of hypoglycemia is factitious use of hypoglycemic agents (insulin or insulin secretagogues (sulfonylureas or meglitinides)). These persons usually have some type of psychiatric problem and derive some secondary gain from these attacks (e.g., sympathy from family, time off from work, etc.). Surreptitious human insulin use can be distinguished from insulinoma by measuring C-peptide levels. Since endogenous insulin is produced by the cleavage of proinsulin to insulin and C-peptide, the plasma levels of both are elevated; with injection of exogenous insulin, only the insulin level is elevated.

However, since many currently prescribed insulins are synthetically modified analogs that may not be detected by conventional assays, this picture has become more clouded as it can be challenging to determine if the suspected abuser has injected insulin or not. Sulfonylureas and meglitinides increase endogenous insulin secretion, so the C-peptide test is not useful in this instance (it will be elevated). Urine or plasma drug tests for secretagogue drugs are important in these cases.

REVIEW QUESTIONS

1. A 32-year-old Caucasian woman comes to the office complaining of a 1-month history of polyuria, polydipsia, and 12-lb weight loss. There is no family history of diabetes, and she did not have gestational diabetes with her two pregnancies (age 26 and 30 years). Your examination reveals a thin, pale woman who appears fatigued but not ill. Serum glucose is 328 mg/dL (18.0 mmol/L), and urine dipstick shows 4+ (strongly positive) glucose. A point-of-care hemoglobin A_{1c} is 10.1% (non-diabetic: <6.5%).
   a. Does this woman have diabetes? Why or why not?
   b. What type of diabetes do you think she has?
   c. How would you differentiate between the different types?
   d. What would be your initial treatment?
   Answers:
   (a) The diagnosis of diabetes mellitus is established by the presence of classic signs and symptoms combined with a serum glucose greater than or equal to 200 mg/dL (11.1 mmol/L). Her hemoglobin A_{1c} is also well above the criteria set for the diagnosis of diabetes (6.5%).
   (b) Given her thin habitus and abrupt onset of symptoms, she most likely has type 1 diabetes. Type 1 DM is most common in Caucasian individuals and is less common in other ethnic groups (e.g., those of Hispanic, Asian, or African-American descent). The lack of GDM with her two pregnancies also is against type 2. Also, while not all patients with type 2 DM are overweight or obese, a family history of the disorder is typical.
   (c) Antibodies against the β cell may be useful. The most commonly useful antibody is anti-GAD-65.

   (d) The only logical choice at this point is insulin, regardless of what type of diabetes she has. Since we have determined that she likely has type 1, this is the best choice. Even with type 2, however, there is no combination of non-insulin agents that will bring her hemoglobin A_{1c} into the normal range.

2. A 58-year-old African-American man comes in for a physical, as he has not been to you in some time. He has no complaints. He is obese (BMI 32.2 kg/m^2) and is found to have a fasting glucose of 132 mg/dL (7.26 mmol/L) as well as a hemoglobin A_{1c} of 6.8%. His mother and maternal aunt both have type 2 diabetes. He has a history of hypertension treated with enalapril, and has normal renal and hepatic function.
   a. Does he have diabetes?
   b. What are some therapeutic options for him?
   Answers:
   (a) He meets the criteria for diabetes with both his fasting glucose ≥126 mg/dL and hemoglobin A_{1c} ≥6.5%. Given his obesity and family history, he most likely has type 2 diabetes.
   (b) Probably the best thing initially would be therapeutic lifestyle changes (TLC), including diet and exercise. Easier said than done, but losing weight would be the best option. If that fails, most would start with metformin therapy initially, as he has normal renal and hepatic function.

3. A 17-year-old girl with a 5-year history of poorly controlled type 1 diabetes and depression presents to the emergency department with somnolence, rapid breathing, and dehydration. On examination

she is found to be hypotensive and has a fruity odor to her breath. Serum glucose is 798 mg/dL (43.9 mmol/L) with 4+ urine ketones. Pregnancy test is negative, and blood and urine tests fail to disclose any infections. She is afebrile.

a. What do you think is going on with this patient?
b. What do you think precipitated it?
c. What would be your therapy? Immediate and long-term?

(a) This is a classic presentation of DKA in a patient with type 1 diabetes. Many fruits (e.g., strawberries, raspberries) owe their characteristic smell to medium-chain ketones or their derivatives, hence the "fruity odor" smell to their breath. Deficiency of insulin has resulted in a "vicious cycle" of catabolism where the body is burning fat (which accumulates in the end product of ketones) since it cannot utilize glucose.

(b) The most common cause of DKA (in the absence of a precipitating cause such as infection) is poor compliance and non-adherence to her insulin regimen. This is especially common in adolescents.

(c) The initial therapy should consist of fluid administration to correct the dehydration. After this has been established, she should be given insulin intravenously. A common error is to give the insulin first. While this may seem intuitively correct, what will happen here is that the insulin will drive glucose into the cells, which will take with it water; this will, in effect, deplete the extracellular volume even further. Insulin should not be given until fluid administration has begun. After the ketoacidosis has resolved, she can be transitioned over to her usual insulin regimen (which she likely had not been taking).

The long-term management of this patient is more challenging. Many studies show that the prevalence of depression in patients with type 1 diabetes is more than twice that in patients without diabetes. This is especially true with adolescents, who are struggling with many physiologic and psychosocial changes. Both she and her family should undergo formal counseling and frequent visits with the diabetes support team in order to avoid these incidents in the future.

4. A 35-year-old woman is seen in the emergency department with recurrent severe hypoglycemia which has been occurring over the last 6 months.

She is found unconscious at home with serum glucose of 34 mg/dL (1.89 mmol/L). Serum insulin level is elevated, and C-peptide level is suppressed. The patient's 13-year-old daughter was diagnosed with type 1 diabetes 1 year ago. After stabilization of her glucose and admission to the hospital for observation, the next best step in management should be:

a. CT of the pancreas to look for insulinoma
b. Urine screen for sulfonylureas
c. Exploratory laparotomy
d. Consultation with a psychiatrist
e. Prolonged fast to provoke further hypoglycemia

(d) This is a classic case of factitious insulin abuse, given that the insulin level is elevated and C-peptide level is suppressed. Often, access to insulin is readily available (e.g., family member who takes insulin). This patient needs counseling with a mental health professional before she does serious harm to herself. (a) and (b) would be appropriate if the C-peptide level was elevated. We would not proceed haphazardly to surgery (c) without further documentation of insulinoma, which is biochemically improbable in this case anyway. Prolonged fasting (e) is sometimes done (in the hospital, of course) to provoke hypoglycemia in patients with suspected insulinoma; again, the biochemical profile is more consistent with factitious insulin use.

5. The most common form of diabetic neuropathy is:
a. Cranial nerve palsy
b. Chronic sensory neuropathy ("stocking feet" distribution)
c. Proximal motor neuropathy (amyotrophy)
d. Diabetic gastroparesis
e. Diabetic sudomotor neuropathy (gustatory sweating)

(b) This is the most common form of diabetic neuropathy. The other types (especially sudomotor autonomic neuropathy) are less common.

6. A 22-year-old Caucasian man is admitted to the hospital for treatment of newly diagnosed diabetes. He presented with nonketotic hyperglycemia and classic symptoms of diabetes. He is thin and without family history of diabetes. After starting insulin, his glucose levels returned to normal and he goes home. Several weeks later he noticed that his glucose levels remained normal even though he forgot to take his insulin several times. The *most likely* explanation for his glucose levels remaining normal despite not taking insulin is:

a. He has MODY (maturity-onset diabetes of the young)

b. He had "glucose toxicity" initially when he was diagnosed and now his β cell function has returned

c. He is going through the "honeymoon period" of type 1 diabetes and his insulin requirements will increase in time

d. He probably does not have diabetes and the diagnosis was a mistake

e. His glucometer is probably broken and he needs a new one

(c) After the initial diagnosis of type 1 diabetes, it is common for some residual insulin secretion to return. This "honeymoon phase" may last for months to sometimes a year or more. The prompt initiation of insulin therapy is important as it may preserve residual insulin secretion (making diabetes easier to control for a time). Glucose toxicity (b) is generally seen in patients with type 2 diabetes and improves after euglycemia is achieved. Monogenic forms of diabetes such as MODY (a) are unlikely in patients with no family history.

Calcium Metabolism

REVIEW

Let us review what we learned in the last lecture. Insulin is an important hormone in glucose metabolism. It is made by pancreatic β cells and is cleaved from a precursor molecule called proinsulin. Glucagon is another hormone of arguably lesser importance in glucose metabolism. Glucagon is made in the α cells and is an antagonist to insulin, and therefore important in recovering from hypoglycemia. Insulin is an anabolic hormone that promotes energy storage while glucagon is catabolic (i.e., it breaks down molecules).

Diabetes mellitus (DM) is a common disorder of glucose metabolism, and may be divided into type 1 and type 2 (although it is a heterogeneous disorder with many phenotypes across the spectrum). Type 1 is usually an autoimmune disease and results from the absence or deficiency of insulin and is more commonly seen in children and young adults, although older individuals can develop type 1. Type 1 can also occur in those who have had pancreatectomy, chronic pancreatitis, or infiltrative pancreatic diseases (e.g., hemochromatosis). These patients require insulin in order to live.

Type 2 diabetes is much more common and is primarily a disorder of insulin resistance in which the body uses insulin ineffectively. Many patients (but not all) with type 2 are overweight or obese. Many noninsulin agents are available for the treatment of type 2 DM (both oral and injectable). Insulin may be required for adequate glucose control in patients with type 2 DM, although it is not immediately necessary for life as with type 1. Prediabetes (impaired glucose tolerance, impaired fasting glucose) is a term used for patients whose blood glucose levels lie in the gray area between normal and high enough to meet the criteria for diabetes. Many of these patients develop diabetes in later life, so intervention and surveillance to prevent diabetic complications is essential.

The insulin resistance and hyperinsulinemia of type 2 diabetes ("metabolic syndrome") are very harmful to the body. These factors contribute to the increased incidence of hypertension, cardiovascular disease, obesity, and hyperlipidemia in patients with type 2 diabetes.

Gestational diabetes is diabetes that occurs during pregnancy. This term usually refers to patients who develop a reversible state of glucose intolerance during the late second to third trimester of gestation, and is due to high concentrations of placental substances such as human chorionic somatomammotropin (human placental lactogen). Many patients can be managed with diet, but some will require insulin. Non-insulin therapies are not approved for gestational diabetes. Glucose tolerance usually returns to normal after delivery, although many of these persons develop type 2 diabetes later in life. Patients with preexisting type 1 and type 2 diabetes also may become pregnant, and good glucose control in all pregnant individuals with diabetes is extremely important to prevent complications.

One of the cornerstones of diabetes management is the self-blood glucose monitor. Patients obtain a sample of capillary blood and place it on a small strip that gives them a glucose reading in seconds. Another important tool in diabetes management is the glycated hemoglobin (HbA$_{1c}$) level. This provides an index of glycemic control over the previous 6 weeks and is a useful adjunct to self-blood glucose monitoring. There is now substantial evidence that good diabetes control helps prevent complications as demonstrated by the DCCT and the UKPDS clinical trials (and several subsequent studies).

Patients with diabetes are prone to develop many complications. These may be divided into the microvascular (small blood vessel) and macrovascular (large blood vessel) syndromes. Diabetic neuropathy is a type of microvascular complication in which nerve cells are damaged. The most common type of diabetic neuropathy results in numbness in both feet. This may result in patients developing ulcers because of lack of sensation. Other types of neuropathy are less common.

Diabetic retinopathy is another form of microvascular disease and is a substantial cause of blindness in society. Non-proliferative retinopathy is less serious and normally requires only routine surveillance. Proliferative retinopathy is more ominous and may lead to bleeding inside the eye, retinal detachment, and blindness. This may be treated by laser photocoagulation of the new blood vessels and surgery if necessary.

Diabetic nephropathy is yet another microvascular complication and is heralded by an increase in the glomerular filtration rate. Elevation of urine microalbumin is seen next, followed by a slow decline in glomerular filtration rate and fixed proteinuria. Diabetic nephropathy may be reversible if detected in the early stages. A minority of patients with diabetic nephropathy will develop end-stage renal disease and require renal replacement therapy (dialysis or renal transplantation). End-stage renal disease is the most expensive complication of diabetes to treat.

Diabetic ketoacidosis occurs in patients with type 1 diabetes who lack adequate insulin to meet metabolic needs. This is a vicious cycle in which the body thinks it is starved because it cannot use glucose, when in fact glucose in the serum is actually quite high. The elevated glucose leads to dehydration because of osmotic diuresis, and catabolic hormones such as glucagon and epinephrine worsen the problem, leading to catabolism of fat and protein and production of ketone bodies and ketoacids. This condition results in death if untreated. Treatment involves intravenous insulin and fluids. Hyperosmolar nonketotic syndrome is similar to ketoacidosis but is usually seen in older individuals without total insulin deficiency. These patients have elevated serum glucose levels but do not develop acidosis.

The only effective therapy for type 1 diabetes is insulin. At this time, insulin must be injected into the body; experimental insulin delivery methods such as inhaled insulin have yielded disappointing results, although new formulations are being evaluated. Trials attempting to prevent type 1 DM also have not been promising. Most patients with type 1 diabetes take a combination of short-acting insulin and long-acting or intermediate-acting insulin.

Insulin pumps are also used for selected patients with type 1 diabetes; an insulin pump is a small external device that delivers insulin continuously to the patient by means of a small plastic catheter. These devices are somewhat complicated and require a great deal of compliance for successful use. Nevertheless, studies show increased glucose control and fewer complications in motivated patients on pump therapy.

Transplants of either a whole pancreas or pancreatic islet cells have been shown to be beneficial in select patients with difficult-to-control diabetes. A disadvantage of this type of therapy is the necessity of taking potent immunosuppressive drugs; the long-term survival rates of these grafts do not approach that for some other organs (e.g., kidney).

Treatment for type 2 diabetes may include diet therapy, oral agents, or insulin. Oral agents may be divided into four different categories. The first includes the insulin secretagogues, such as the sulfonylureas and meglitinides. These agents increase insulin secretion by the pancreas and, therefore, can potentially cause hypoglycemia. All other types of oral agents do not, by themselves, cause hypoglycemia (although they can potentiate agents that can). Metformin is a biguanide derivative that decreases hepatic glucose output and increases insulin sensitivity. A very rare side effect of this medication is lactic acidosis that occurs rarely in patients with renal and/or hepatic insufficiency; this is not a consideration if appropriately prescribed. The thiazolidinediones are novel drugs that increase insulin sensitivity. Relatively new drugs such as DPP-IV inhibitors and GLP-1 antagonists improve gastric emptying and improve insulin sensitivity. SGLUT inhibitors such as canagliflozin inhibit renal reabsorption of glucose. Finally, α-glucosidase inhibitors decrease absorption of disaccharides and small polysaccharides by the small intestine, leading to decreased glucose levels after meals.

Hypoglycemia is a disorder that, while perpetuated by the media as a cause of many ills, is actually quite rare. It was believed in the past to be quite common, probably due to overuse of the glucose tolerance test. True reactive hypoglycemia is actually quite rare in the absence of structural gastrointestinal tract abnormalities. Insulinoma is a pathological cause of hypoglycemia—patients have spontaneous hypoglycemia and may develop seizures and even die if untreated. Another important cause of hypoglycemia is the factitious use of insulin and oral hypoglycemic agents, seen sometimes in patients with psychiatric disorders. Laboratory studies sometimes can help distinguish between endogenous and factitious causes of hypoglycemia, although the widespread use of synthetic insulin analogs (some of which are not detected by insulin assays) has made this evaluation more complex.

TRANSPORT AND REGULATION OF CALCIUM

Although calcium lacks the glamour of the other hormones, it is important in many processes, including muscle contraction, synaptic transmission in the nervous system, platelet aggregation, coagulation, and secretion of hormones (as an intracellular second messenger). Unlike most of the hormones we have discussed, it is not under direct control by the pituitary gland or hypothalamus and is to some extent like the "special team" squad on our football team.

Like iodothyronine hormones and sex steroids, the divalent cation calcium travels bound to serum proteins (such as albumin). About one-half is bound to proteins or other substances, while the remaining half circulates as free (commonly called "ionized") calcium. Like other hormones, it is the free, or unbound, moiety that is biologically active.

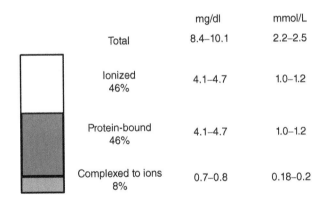

	mg/dl	mmol/L
Total	8.4–10.1	2.2–2.5
Ionized 46%	4.1–4.7	1.0–1.2
Protein-bound 46%	4.1–4.7	1.0–1.2
Complexed to ions 8%	0.7–0.8	0.18–0.2

Ionized calcium = active form

Total calcium is influenced by amount of serum proteins

Corrected Ca^{2+} = Measured Ca^{2+} + (0.8)(4 − serum albumin)

Calcium in Plasma

Calcium is not a "classical" hormone since it is not secreted from a gland; instead, it comes from several different sources. The largest supply of calcium is the skeleton, which houses over 99% of the body's calcium as a calcium phosphate salt. Dietary calcium also may be absorbed by the small intestine. The kidney plays an important role in reabsorbing calcium that is present in the blood and filtered through the urinary system. Adequate calcium intake (1,000–1,500 mg elemental calcium/day) is recommended for normal health. It is important that you understand that patients need the recommended amount of *elemental* calcium and not just the mass of the salt. For example, calcium carbonate (the most common preparation) is 40% elemental calcium by mass; therefore, one must take 2,500 mg of calcium carbonate to receive 1,000 of elemental calcium per day. Calcium citrate, however, is only 20% elemental calcium by mass; 5,000 mg of the citrate salt is required to obtain 1,000 mg elemental calcium.

The primary regulator of calcium metabolism is parathyroid hormone (PTH), secreted by the parathyroid glands. These small but mighty glands are pea sized and usually located posterior to the thyroid gland. Most people have four parathyroids, but occasionally people have fewer or greater. An occasional individual may have a parathyroid located in another location, such as the mediastinum.

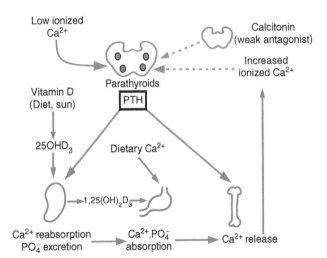

Regulation of Calcium Metabolism

When serum calcium becomes low, this signals an increase in PTH levels. This process is mediated by the extracellular calcium-sensing receptor (CaSR). There are three actions of PTH that help restore serum calcium to normal:

1. Increased resorption of calcium from bone.
2. Increased reabsorption of calcium from the kidney.
3. Increased calcium absorption from the intestine.

PTH has no direct effect on dietary calcium absorption. It indirectly increases absorption due to its ability to increase the concentration of active vitamin D metabolites (via its effect on the kidney, which facilitates conversion of vitamin D to calcitriol).

When calcium and PTH levels are normal, PTH actually enhances formation of bone. It is only with pathological elevation of PTH levels that pathologic bone resorption occurs.

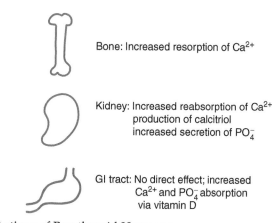

Bone: Increased resorption of Ca^{2+}

Kidney: Increased reabsorption of Ca^{2+}
production of calcitriol
increased secretion of PO_4^-

GI tract: No direct effect; increased
Ca^{2+} and PO_4^- absorption
via vitamin D

Actions of Parathyroid Hormone

Vitamin D is also important in calcium metabolism. It is derived from cholesterol and is a sterol hormone formed from photogenesis in the skin and absorption from food. Vitamin D_2 (ergocalciferol) is obtained from eating plants and fungi (produced by photoconversion of precursors in those organisms), while vitamin D_3 (cholecalciferol) is formed in animals by the photoconversion of sterol precursors found in the skin, such as 7-dehydrocholesterol; they are of similar activity, and will simply be referred to as vitamin D here.

Vitamin D was discovered in 1924, when scientists found that irradiation of an animal or its food prevented rickets. Even a small amount of sun exposure is enough to ensure adequate vitamin D stores in most persons (excessive sun exposure is obviously not recommended given the increased risk of skin cancer). Vitamin D itself has little activity but is converted to various activated metabolites. One of the major ones is calcidiol. The most important step in vitamin D metabolism is the conversion of calcidiol to calcitriol in the kidney. Calcitriol is the most active metabolite of vitamin D $(1,25(OH)_2D)$ and its primary effect is increasing calcium and phosphorus absorption in the intestine. Vitamin D receptors are present in many other organs and the vitamin's immense role in other processes is continually being investigated; it appears to play a role in immune modulation and may even have a role in glucose homeostasis, among other things. Hypocalcemia increases and hypercalcemia inhibits synthesis of calcitriol. The recommended dose of vitamin D for most adults is 600–800 units daily.

Calcitonin is a small protein secreted by the parafollicular (C) cells of the thyroid (as opposed to T4 and T3, which are made in the follicular cells). It is a weak antagonist of PTH and is secreted in response to hypercalcemia. Calcitonin is very important in salt water animals (e.g., fish, eels) that live in a high-calcium environment such as the ocean, but its importance is negligible in humans (we know this since removal of the thyroid gland has no significant effect on bone metabolism in humans).

HYPERCALCEMIA

Mild hypercalcemia may present without symptoms. Moderate to severe hypercalcemia usually presents with symptoms of neuromuscular suppression. In general, symptoms include dehydration, weight loss, anorexia, pruritus, and polydipsia. Patients may also present with nausea, vomiting, fatigue, lethargy, confusion, and in severe cases, coma. Next, we will explore the various causes of hypercalcemia.

Hyperparathyroidism

The most common cause of hypercalcemia in the asymptomatic adult is primary hyperparathyroidism, with an incidence of about 1 in 800 patients. Most patients are asymptomatic and are detected only through routine screening. This condition results when one or more abnormally functioning glands secrete too much PTH, which causes increased reabsorption of calcium by the kidney, increased release of calcium by bone, and increased calcium absorption from the intestine (indirectly via vitamin D). Because increased PTH levels cause increased phosphate excretion (phosphaturia), serum phosphorus is decreased.

Most cases of primary hyperparathyroidism (about 80%) are due to a solitary parathyroid adenoma.

The rest are usually due to hyperplasia of all four glands. Parathyroid carcinoma is a very rare and aggressive form of hyperparathyroidism.

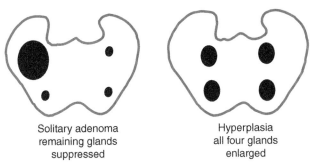

Solitary adenoma
remaining glands
suppressed

Hyperplasia
all four glands
enlarged

Primary Hyperparathyroidism

At this time, surgery remains the most effective treatment for primary hyperparathyroidism. Not everyone needs to be treated, though. Indications for treating primary hyperparathyroidism include serum calcium >1.0 mg/dL (0.25 mmol/L) over the normal upper limit (usually about 10.2 mg/dL (2.55 mmol/L)); osteoporosis (DEXA T score ≤ -2.5 at any site, and/or presence of fragility fracture); age less than 50 years; reduced creatinine clearance (<60 mL/min). (Previously, 24-h urine calcium excretion >400 mg was an indication, but this criterion has been removed.) Patients who do not meet these criteria can simply be monitored on an annual basis, although the ultimate decision must be tailored to the individual patient.

What is a fragility fracture? A fragility fracture results from mechanical stress forces that would not ordinarily result in fracture, known as low-energy trauma. The World Health Organization (WHO) has quantified this as "forces equivalent to a fall from a standing height or less." For example, an elderly woman who fractures her radius after falling on her living room carpet has suffered a fragility fracture while a 320-lb pro football guard who fractures his radius after smashing into the opponents' defensive line has not.

One might logically think that restriction of calcium intake would be advised in this disorder. While excessive calcium supplementation is not recommended, restriction of calcium intake may actually worsen the hyperparathyroidism, and 1,000 mg/day of elemental calcium is recommended for most patients with primary HPT. Adequate vitamin D intake (400–600 units daily) is also desired.

A novel calcimimetic agent, cinacalcet, activates the parathyroid CaSR and "fools" the parathyroids into thinking the calcium level is even higher, which can decrease secretion. Why does this work? Remember that most benign endocrine tumors exhibit some feedback inhibition from the excess target hormone; an example we studied earlier was Cushing's disease. The false sense of "higher" calcium levels can result in some regression of the benign tumor. Since this medication is expensive and not a cure for the problem, it is reserved for those patients in whom treatment is indicated and who refuse surgical treatment and/or are poor surgical risks. The treatment of choice for primary hyperparathyroidism is, again, surgical excision of one or more abnormal parathyroid glands. In patients with a solitary adenoma, it is removed. In hyperplasia, the majority of all four glands are removed. Patients with asymptomatic disease and minimal calcium elevation often do not require surgery (see recommendations above).

If surgery has been elected, several localization procedures may be useful prior to the procedure. At this time, the best test utilizes a combination of ultrasound and technetium-labeled sestamibi, a substance often used in nuclear cardiology. This procedure helps the surgeon localize the abnormal parathyroid gland(s) prior to surgery, which may decrease surgical time. Like a thyroid scan, it is not a diagnostic test; the diagnosis still relies on serum biochemistry.

Patients with renal insufficiency may develop a different type of hyperparathyroidism. These patients often develop hypocalcemia because of decreased calcium reabsorption, chronic phosphate retention, and diminished production of calcitriol. This long-standing hypocalcemia results in elevated PTH levels that have no effect on the kidney, but still have effect on bone. Over time, these elevated PTH levels can cause bone resorption and bone pain. Treatment requires restriction of dietary phosphate, phosphate-binding agents, and calcitriol to help increase the serum calcium. Cinacalcet is often used in this disorder to suppress PTH levels. Since the hyperparathyroidism has been precipitated by another cause, it is called secondary hyperparathyroidism.

If this condition progresses too long, the parathyroid gland hypersecretion becomes autonomous and persists even after calcium is brought into the normal range. This is called tertiary hyperparathyroidism and is difficult to manage. In this disorder, the only current therapy is removal of most of the parathyroid glands, since secretion is autonomous and generally does not respond to calcimimetic agents such as cinacalcet.

Malignancy-associated hypercalcemia

Most patients with severe hypercalcemia have cancer, and the most common cause of malignancy-related hypercalcemia is humoral hypercalcemia of malignancy (HHM). The most common specific tumor type is squamous cell lung carcinoma, although other adenocarcinomas (such as breast carcinoma, renal cell carcinoma, and bladder carcinoma) may also be causes. We usually associate ectopic endocrine syndromes with small cell lung cancer (not squamous), but in fact small cell cancer does not produce hypercalcemia. Tumors causing HHM secrete PTH-related peptide (PTH-rP), which acts in a manner similar to PTH. PTH-rP is present in small amounts in normal persons and is necessary for development of cartilage cells, mammary glands, hair follicles, and skin; in fact, it appears to be the "PTH" of the fetus (levels of PTH-rP rarely may increase sufficiently in pregnancy to cause transient hypercalcemia). Patients with pathological PTH-rP secretion, however, have laboratory findings similar to patients with hyperparathyroidism: hypercalcemia with hypophosphatemia. Native PTH secretion is inhibited by hypercalcemia, so PTH levels are low in non-PTH-mediated hypercalcemia.

Local osteolytic hypercalcemia (LOH) is a less common cause of tumor-associated hypercalcemia. This disorder is due to secretion of substances called osteoclast activating factors (OAFs), and not by direct tumor invasion by bone. Examples include breast cancer and multiple myeloma. Some examples of these substances include PTHrp, interleukins, transforming growth factors (TGFs), prostaglandins, and procathepsin D.

Vitamin D-dependent hypercalcemia

Hypercalcemia may also occur if excess vitamin D is present. The manufacture of vitamin D is tightly regulated by feedback inhibition, so synthesis of the active metabolites (e.g., calcitriol) is usually shut off when ordinary vitamin D (e.g., from multivitamins) is ingested. Vitamin D toxicity may occur when high-potency pharmacologic preparations (e.g., calcitriol) are ingested; it is less likely to occur with over-the-counter preparations (ergocalciferol, cholecalciferol) unless very high doses are ingested, but this does occur on occasion.

Granulomatous diseases (such as tuberculosis, sarcoidosis, berylliosis, and leprosy) may also cause vitamin D-dependent hypercalcemia. The cells of these lesions may possess the enzyme necessary to convert more primitive vitamin D forms to calcitriol, resulting in hypercalcemia. Some hematologic malignancies such as lymphomas produce extra vitamin D, and may be considered a paraneoplastic syndrome (to be discussed further in the last lecture).

The treatment of vitamin D-dependent hypercalcemia obviously involves removal of the vitamin D source, if present. Treatment of the systemic diseases mentioned above is important. Glucocorticoids are a mainstay of treatment because they decrease calcium absorption from the intestine and result in a prompt decrease in calcium levels.

Other causes

Some endocrine disorders also may cause hypercalcemia. Hyperthyroidism may lead to increased bone resorption of calcium. This form of hypercalcemia is usually mild, with few or no symptoms, and responds promptly to treatment of hyperthyroidism. Persistence of hypercalcemia after treatment suggests another cause.

Adrenal insufficiency also may cause mild hypercalcemia. This condition is aggravated by the dehydration that normally occurs during adrenal insufficiency. Rehydration and steroid replacement promptly restore calcium levels to normal.

Milk-alkali syndrome may occur after the ingestion of large amounts of calcium (e.g., milk) and alkali (e.g., sodium bicarbonate), usually taken for a peptic ulcer or esophagitis. The metabolic alkalosis results in hypocalciuria and later, hypercalcemia. Renal failure often occurs. This disorder is uncommon today because of vastly improved treatments of peptic ulcer disease (i.e., proton pump inhibitors), and at one time was felt to be an extinct entity. It was much more common in the past, when ulcer patients drank whole bottles of milk along with boxes of baking soda ($NaHCO_3$) to relieve their ailment. Recently, however, there has been resurgence in the use of calcium for prevention of osteoporosis. Some patients consume more than the prescribed amount of calcium (often due to increasing varieties of flavored tablets), resulting in more cases of this syndrome in recent years.

Hypercalcemic crisis

Hypercalcemic crisis is the end stage of hypercalcemia, and may lead to coma and death. Although any of the above conditions can cause it, it usually is associated with malignancy. Since these patients are usually severely dehydrated (calcium acts as an osmotic diuretic), the most important first step is rehydration with intravenous fluids. After rehydration has been established, loop diuretics (furosemide) promote calciuria, and are especially useful in those with renal failure. Doing this backwards (giving the diuretics before adequate hydration has been established) will invariably make the condition worse.

Glucocorticoids are useful in the vitamin D-dependent hypercalcemias, hypercalcemia of adrenal insufficiency, and hypercalcemia associated with certain osteolytic tumors and hematologic malignancies, but are of minimal use in other conditions. HHM is best treated with an antiresorptive agent. These include parenteral potent bisphosphonates (zoledronic acid and pamidronate), which bind irreversibly to bone and prevent its resorption. Salmon calcitonin has mild antiresorptive action and may be useful in mild hypercalcemia. After calcium levels have returned to normal, treatment of the underlying disease (e.g., malignancy) is indicated.

HYPOCALCEMIA

While hypercalcemia causes neuromuscular suppression, hypocalcemia results in neuromuscular excitability. Typical manifestations include paresthesias (numbness and tingling (typically in the hands and around the mouth)), hyperventilation, tetany, adrenergic symptoms (e.g., tachycardia, diaphoresis), seizures, Chvostek's and Trousseau's signs, QT interval prolongation, hypotension, refractory CHF, cardiomegaly, abnormalities in dental formation, gastrointestinal malabsorption, and cataracts.

Chvostek's and Trousseau's signs may be seen in those with hypocalcemia and latent tetany. Chvostek's sign is elicited by tapping the face in the area of the facial nerve. A positive response elicits spasm of the facial muscles on that side. Many normal persons have a slight Chvostek's sign. Trousseau's sign is elicited by inflating a blood pressure cuff around the arm between systolic and diastolic blood pressures. This is continued for several minutes, and the time to carpal spasm is noted, if positive.

Hypocalcemia may be caused by many conditions. Just as hypercalcemia can be caused by too much PTH, hypocalcemia may occur if there is not enough. This condition is called hypoparathyroidism and the most common cause is inadvertent surgical damage or removal (e.g., from removal of the thyroid). It also may be present for no apparent reason (idiopathic). In addition to hypocalcemia, hyperphosphatemia may be present, since PTH normally promotes phosphorus excretion by the body.

Persons with hypoparathyroidism have low calcium levels, because PTH effects on bone and kidney are diminished. Hyperphosphatemia is present, since PTH normally causes phosphate excretion by the kidney. PTH levels are of course diminished.

The treatment of hypoparathyroidism is one example where the native hormone is not normally used as a replacement. This means that its effects on the two major sites—kidney and bone—are lost forever. Its third effect (that of enhancing calcitriol production) can be mimicked by administering calcitriol or other vitamin D analogs orally. With sufficient doses and dietary calcium supplementation, serum calcium levels return to normal.

Synthetic (1–34) PTH has been available as a treatment for osteoporosis for several years; it is being studied in clinical trials as a potential therapy for hypoparathyroidism. A potential benefit is decreased excretion of calcium. Disadvantages include the need for injection and the very high cost when compared to vitamin D therapy. Also, the long-term effects of 1–34 PTH on the skeleton are unknown; currently, lifetime duration of therapy for osteoporosis is limited to 2 years.

Another condition similar to hypoparathyroidism occurs when the body is resistant to PTH action. This produces a clinical picture similar to hypoparathyroidism, except that the PTH levels are elevated. This syndrome is called pseudohypoparathyroidism (false hypoparathyroidism). In addition to the hypocalcemia and hyperphosphatemia, these patients often have some characteristic clinical features: short stature, obesity, short fourth metacarpals (brachydactyly), and mental retardation. The treatment of pseudohypoparathyroidism is similar to that of hypoparathyroidism (vitamin D analogs plus calcium supplementation).

You might ask an obvious question: can hypocalcemia not occur because of dietary deficiency? (This can happen with most other substances in the body (iron, magnesium, vitamins, etc.).) But, this is virtually impossible with calcium, because the skeleton contains vast amounts of calcium, which is adequate to keep calcium levels normal (even in the face of dietary deficiency). In nutritional deficiency, the cost is, however, loss of bone, leading to osteoporosis. Adequate calcium (and vitamin D) intake is important for normal bone mass, especially during the adolescent years, when bone growth velocity is at its highest.

A good way to help determine the etiology of hyper- or hypocalcemia is to plot the serum calcium concentration against the PTH level. This helps divide the values into four categories: low calcium, low PTH; low calcium, high PTH; high calcium, high PTH; and high calcium, low PTH.

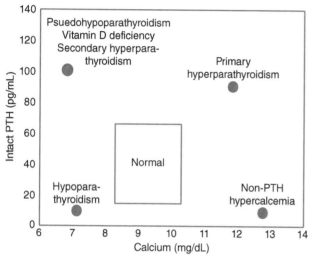

Graph of Serum Calcium versus PTH Level in Various Calcium Disorders

BONE

Bone provides rigid support and protection for extremities and body cavities containing vital organs, and provides effective levers for muscles. It also has a metabolic function, serving as a large reservoir of ions (calcium, magnesium, and phosphorus). Without bone, we would simply be a large mass of organic protoplasm quivering on the floor. A marvel of evolutionary engineering, it provides enormous support and strength while being relatively lightweight.

There are two major types of bone. Cortical or compact bone is found in tubular bones (e.g., radius, tibia). Trabecular or cancellous bone is found in the vertebrae and axial skeleton.

Bone is more than just a hard structure that supports our tissues; it is a living organ that is constantly being remodeled. It consists of a matrix (collagenous proteins that form the framework) and minerals (calcium salts laid over the matrix). The molecules in your femur today are not the same as 3 years ago. Normally, the amount resorbed equals the amount formed; osteoblasts form new bone on the surface and synthesize new matrix (collagenous proteins). Osteocytes are merely osteoblasts after they are trapped in mineralized matrix. Osteoclasts are multinucleated giant cells involved in bone resorption.

Osteoporosis

Osteoporosis is the condition of a decreased quantity of bone (mineralization + matrix). Osteoporosis is a major public health problem that is responsible for over 2 million fractures and over $20 billion in direct health care costs in the United States each year. One in two women over the age of 50 and one in eight men over age 50 will have an osteoporosis-related fracture in their lifetime.

The pathogenesis of osteoporosis involves uncoupling of the normal balance between bone formation and resorption. The bone present is structurally normal, but of reduced quantity. In normal health, the amount formed equals amount resorbed. In osteoporosis, either too much bone is resorbed (high turnover) or too little is formed (low turnover).

What are some risk factors for osteoporosis? Genetics obviously plays a role; like most disorders, patients are more likely to have osteoporosis if they have a strong family history. Certain ethnic groups are more likely to develop osteoporosis. Traditionally, those of northern European and Asian descent are more likely to develop osteoporosis than other groups. African Americans, conversely, have the highest bone density among ethnic groups. Patients who are overweight are less likely to develop osteoporosis (at least one positive thing about being overweight!). Overweight persons may have increased bone mass compared to normal people because of the stress on the bones of carrying extra weight around (but remember the stress energy is greater in their falls due to the higher mass). Cigarette smoking is a risk factor for osteoporosis, as is excess alcohol consumption. Immobilization is another risk factor; patients who are bedridden for a long time eventually lose a great deal of bone mass. Space scientists discovered that astronauts in a weightless environment lost a tremendous amount of bone density unless they engaged in regular exercise aboard the spacecraft. Without adequate exercise, an astronaut taking a 1-year-long trip to Mars would break his or her legs after stepping onto the Martian surface merely from the loss of bone mass during the trip (despite its gravity being only 0.38 that of Earth).

The most frequent cause of osteoporosis in women is postmenopausal. Most bone loss occurs within the first 5–10 years after menopause or oophorectomy, and is a "high turnover" form of osteoporosis (estrogen deficiency accelerates bone resorption). But not all postmenopausal patients develop osteoporosis—it is important to identify those patients at risk and treat as soon as possible. Given the potential health risks of estrogen, however, this therapy is reserved only for selected individuals, as other agents are available. Those menopausal women with normal or high bone density can simply be monitored (while taking the recommended calcium and vitamin D supplementation). But estrogen is still an excellent treatment for certain patients.

Corticosteroids are the most common cause of drug-induced osteoporosis, since they are used for many chronic diseases. Since they inhibit bone formation, this is a low turnover form of osteoporosis.

Osteoporosis is less common in men, because they start out with higher bone mass than women, and do not have an abrupt decline in gonadal steroids in mid-life as women do (menopause). Men with testosterone deficiency (hypogonadism) may develop osteoporosis, especially if it occurs in early adulthood.

Osteoporosis is a straightforward diagnosis for patients with obvious osteopenia on X-ray and pathologic fractures (e.g., compression fracture of the spine). Plain X-rays, however, are usually a poor method of diagnosing osteoporosis in its early stages because a tremendous amount of bone must be lost before it can be reliably detected by this method. The test of choice is dual-energy X-ray absorptiometry (DEXA), which is noninvasive, has high precision/accuracy, and is easy to perform.

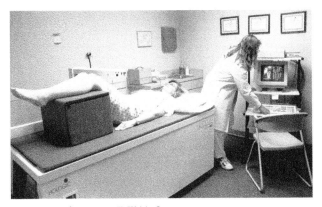

Patient Undergoing DEXA Scan

Bone density is typically measured in the lumbar spine and femoral neck, and plotted on a graph. The values are compared to others in his/her age group and to young adults. It has been found that fracture correlates best when compared to young adults (peak bone mass) than with others the same age. For example, a 95-year-old woman with a bone density at the 75th percentile for her age still has significant risk of fracture since virtually all persons this age have osteoporosis (by DEXA definition).

Bone density, like most human measurements, is normally distributed. Persons with a bone density greater than the 16th percentile (greater than one standard deviation below the mean) for young adults are said to have normal bone density. Those with bone density between −2.5 and −1.0 standard deviations below the mean have low bone mass or osteopenia. Those with a value less than 2.5 standard deviations below the mean (<2 percentile) have osteoporosis. Is osteopenia (low bone mass) a disease? Not necessarily; like most things in medicine, the measurement must be put in proper clinical context. Just as not everyone is tall, not everyone has a high bone density; someone has to be below the mean. Smaller people, on average, have lower bone densities, proportional to their mass. Risk of fracture is also relative, and patients with low bone densities may never have fractures if they are sedentary. On the other hand, any bone can fracture, given sufficient stress; 300-lb pro football linemen with very high bone densities routinely suffer fractures after smashing into each other on Sunday afternoons (remember our discussion of "fragility fractures").

Laboratory studies of people with osteoporosis are typically normal. However, screening to exclude secondary causes should be considered in many patients to exclude metabolic disease. Primary hyperparathyroidism is one cause of osteoporosis that is correctable.

Treatment of osteoporosis

There are many treatments for osteoporosis. In patients with hypogonadism, it is usually desirable to replace the sex steroids. The first decision is whether to treat or not. Patients with DEXA criteria for osteoporosis (T score ≤ −2.5) are treated, as are those with established fragility fractures. Patients with osteopenia (T score between −1 and −2.5) are not necessarily treated. In postmenopausal or oophorectomized women in whom it is not contraindicated (those with breast cancer or active thromboembolic disease), estrogen is an option, although much less commonly used today given its potential adverse health effects. Estrogen, if used, is much more effective if started soon after menopause or oophorectomy, since most bone is lost during the first 5 years after menopause or oophorectomy. Men with hypogonadism should receive androgen therapy unless contraindicated (e.g., prostate cancer).

Bisphosphonates (already discussed with treatment of hypercalcemia) are phosphate analogs that bind to bone, thus preventing resorption. They have minimal effect on bone formation. Alendronate, risedronate, and ibandronate are oral bisphosphonates used for osteoporosis. Zoledronic acid is an intravenous bisphosphonate that has the advantage of once-yearly administration.

While generally well tolerated, the bisphosphonates have been associated with rare yet debilitating side effects. One rare side effect is that of osteonecrosis of the jaw; those who have undergone recent dental surgery are at higher risk. Another is atypical femoral fractures (AFF), which differ from typical osteoporotic femoral fractures in many respects, including the mechanism of injury, location, and fracture configuration. The risk appears to be higher with zoledronic acid. With evidence of little benefit when used for more than 5 years (oral bisphosphonates) or 3 years (intravenous zoledronic acid) and given the potential serious adverse events, it may be appropriate to stop treatment after this interval in most patients and re-evaluate.

Salmon calcitonin also inhibits bone resorption and has an analgesic effect. It is available either as a subcutaneous form or as a nasal spray. Raloxifene is a synthetic estrogen receptor modulator (SERM) that may be given to certain patients who cannot tolerate estrogen or in whom estrogen is contraindicated (e.g.,

breast cancer survivors). It has the antiresorptive properties of estrogen but no other hormonal effects, so it is not useful in preventing symptoms such as vasomotor flashes. SERMs also slightly increase the risk of venous thromboembolism.

Denosumab is a novel monoclonal antibody (administered subcutaneously) against the RANK ligand (inhibition of this receptor inhibits osteoclasts and therefore bone resorption); it is given as a single subcutaneous injection once every 6 months. As with other immunotherapies, it has been associated with an increased risk of infection.

Teriparatide (1–34 synthetic PTH) also stimulates bone formation in many patients (it is the only anabolic therapy for osteoporosis; the others are antiresorptive); it can only be given for a total of 2 years (lifetime dose) and is contraindicated in patients with a history of radiation therapy. It is given by daily subcutaneous injection.

Calcium and vitamin D supplementation are recommended in all patients as well as healthy adults (there is some evidence that calcium without vitamin D may actually be harmful, though). Risks for osteoporosis (smoking, corticosteroid use, high-fall risk living environment, etc.) should be reduced or eliminated if possible.

Agents Used for the Therapy of Osteoporosis

Agent	Method of Administration	Action	Notes
Calcium/vitamin D	Oral	Necessary for normal bone formation in all humans	Indicated for all patients (including healthy adults)
Estrogen	Oral, transdermal	Antiresorptive	Increased risk of breast cancer, cardiovascular disease, thromboembolic events
Bisphosphonates (alendronate, risedronate, ibandronate, zoledronic acid)	Oral, intravenous (zoledronic acid)	Antiresorptive	Increased risk of esophageal irritation, osteonecrosis of jaw, and atypical femoral fractures with long-term use
Monoclonal antibody (denosumab)	Subcutaneous injection	Antiresorptive	Increased risk of infections, rash, joint pain
Teriparatide	Subcutaneous injection	Anabolic	Contraindicated in patients with history of radiation; lifetime duration of therapy 2 years maximum
Selective estrogen-receptor modulator (raloxifene)	Oral	Antiresorptive	Increased risk of thromboembolic events
Salmon calcitonin	Subcutaneous injection or nasal spray	Antiresorptive	May have additional analgesic effects.

So, who should be treated with these agents, since most are associated with potentially serious side effects? Those with osteoporosis by DEXA (*T* score −2.5 or less) are candidates for treatment, as are those with a fragility fracture (regardless of BMD). Those with low bone mass or osteopenia (*T* score between −1.0 and −2.5) are treated if they are at high risk. The WHO's FRAX (Fracture Risk Assessment) is an online tool that yields a person's 10-year probability of fracture; the tool is normalized to specific continents and ethnic populations. The tool takes into account many risk factors in addition to the DEXA T score (e.g., smoking history, alcohol use, family history, corticosteroid use, etc.). In the United States, it is recommended that patients with osteopenia be treated if the 10-year probability of a major osteoporosis-related fracture is at least 20% or at least 3% for a hip fracture. It must be emphasized that the FRAX tool is merely a recommendation and the decision whether to treat is ultimately up to the provider and the patient.

VITAMIN D DEFICIENCY

Many people receive inadequate sun exposure to provide adequate vitamin D levels; therefore mild vitamin D deficiency is relatively common. They often do not receive adequate dietary intake, and conditions such as obesity appear to predispose to vitamin D deficiency.

Osteomalacia

Osteomalacia is another disorder of calcium metabolism that is biochemically distinct from osteoporosis. In osteoporosis, both calcification and organic matrix are deficient. In osteomalacia, the organic matrix is normal, but calcification is deficient. When osteomalacia occurs in children, it is called rickets.

Patients with osteomalacia commonly develop deformities caused by fractures in ribs, vertebrae, and long bones, and often have a '"waddling gait" with muscle weakness and diffuse skeletal pain. A classic radiologic finding is the presence of a radiolucent band (called psuedofractures or Looser's zones), often in the long bones, metatarsals, pelvis, and scapula.

The etiology of osteomalacia is usually from vitamin D deficiency, which leads to hypocalcemia and hypophosphatemia. Less commonly, metabolic errors in calcium and/or phosphorus metabolism can cause this disorder. Drugs such as some anticonvulsants may interfere with vitamin D metabolism and cause osteomalacia. Serum calcidiol are typically low, and PTH levels are increased if the patient has hypocalcemia. Alkaline phosphatase (a marker of bone formation) is usually elevated.

The treatment of osteomalacia includes vitamin D analogs (e.g., calcitriol), dietary calcium, and phosphate, which restore calcium and phosphorus levels to normal. Malabsorption also should be treated, if present. Tumor-associated osteomalacia is an interesting condition in which osteomalacia appears to be caused by some type of humoral factor secreted by the tumor. This disorder improves with treatment of the malignancy.

Paget's disease of bone

Finally, let us discuss another type of disorder called Paget's disease, which is basically an error in bone remodeling. In normal bone, bone formation equals bone resorption at all sites. In Paget's disease, however, excessive resorption and formation occur at different sites, resulting in a disorganized mosaic of bone at affected sites. It is a common disorder, although many cases go undiagnosed because of the lack of symptoms.

Most patients are asymptomatic and discovered incidentally by X-ray, bone scan, or elevated alkaline phosphatase level. Few patients present with pain directly related to the pagetic process. Bowing deformities of the limbs can lead to pain, shortened limbs, and gait abnormalities. The normal side may be affected by abnormal weight bearing. Osteoarthritis is a common secondary complication, and it may be difficult to separate this from pagetic pain.

Since Paget's disease is a disorder of bone remodeling, it may be treated by agents such as bisphosphonates (alendronate, zoledronic acid) with satisfactory results in most cases. Rarely, pagetic bone may transition into osteosarcoma, an especially ominous disorder of bone.

REVIEW QUESTIONS

1. A 57-year-old woman is seen by her primary care physician for a routine examination. Serum calcium level drawn at a health fair is 10.9 mg/dL (normal: 8.4–10.2); the repeat value is 11.0 mg/dL. Serum PTH level is modestly elevated at 88 pg/mL (N: 6–56), and serum phosphorus is low normal at 2.8 mg/dL. The patient is asymptomatic and has no history of kidney stones or fractures. A recent DEXA scan shows normal bone density in the spine, femoral neck, and radius.
   a. What is the likely diagnosis?
   b. What should the treatment be?
   (a) The diagnosis likely is primary hyperparathyroidism, a common diagnosis (1 in 800 women).
   (b) This patient falls into the category of "asymptomatic" hyperparathyroidism and meets no criteria for surgery (calcium >1.0 mg/dL above normal, kidney stones, presence of osteoporosis, young age).

2. A 47-year-old woman presents to the emergency department one day after undergoing a total thyroidectomy for papillary thyroid cancer with complaints of muscle cramps and tingling in her hands and around her mouth. Chvostek's sign is strongly positive, and serum calcium is low at 6.4 mg/dL (8.4–10.2), with high normal phosphorus of 4.5 mg/dL (2.8–4.5).
   a. What is the likely diagnosis?
   b. What would be the initial treatment?
   c. What is the long-term treatment?
   (a) She likely has postsurgical hypoparathyroidism, an inadvertent complication of her thyroidectomy.
   (b) The most important initial therapy is the administration of intravenous calcium as a continuous infusion. Oral calcium would not be effective in this setting.
   (c) It is possible that the hypoparathyroidism is transient and may resolve; however, it is prudent to begin therapy with potent vitamin D analogs (calcitriol) and oral calcium supplementation. Synthetic PTH (teriparatide) is being studied as a therapy for hypoparathyroidism, but its expense and long-term side effects are potential issues (it is only approved for a duration of 2 years when used for osteoporosis). Most patients are easily controlled with vitamin D analogs and calcium, despite the fact that this replaces only one component of PTH action (the renal and bone effects are lost).

3. A 23-year-old female is seen for hypocalcemia (6.7 mg/dL (N: 8.2–10.4 mg/dL). Ionized calcium is checked and is also low. Serum phosphorus is high at 5.2 mg/dL (N: 2.5–5.2 mg/dL). Physical examination reveals short stature (59 in. (150 cm)) and hands with short third fingers, which are shorter than the index fingers. Serum PTH is three times normal. The patient was not able to complete high school due to academic deficiencies and is asymptomatic. What is the most likely diagnosis?
   a. Dietary calcium deficiency
   b. Psuedohypoparathyroidism
   c. Hypoparathyroidism
   d. Excess ingestion of phosphate-containing antacids
   (b) This is a classic presentation of pseudohypoparathyroidism with mild mental retardation, short stature, brachydactyly (short third metacarpals), and resistance to PTH. It can be distinguished from hypoparathyroidism because of the high PTH level (low in (c)). Dietary calcium deficiency does not cause hypocalcemia.

4. A 68-year-old woman presents for a routine health maintenance examination, which includes a DEXA scan. She has no fracture history, but her mother fractured her hip at age 63. She does smoke cigarettes but does not take glucocorticoids and does not drink alcohol. Her femoral neck BMD is 0.701 g/cm², which provides a FRAX 10-year probability of fracture of 17% (major osteoporotic) and 4.6% (hip fracture). She currently has no health problems, is asymptomatic, and takes no medications. What recommendations would you give for this patient, in addition to recommending she quit smoking and adding calcium and vitamin D supplementation?
   a. Estrogen
   b. Oral alendronate, once weekly
   c. Observation
   d. Denosumab
   e. Teriparatide

(b) This patient is at high risk for hip fracture given her FRAX probability of 4.6% (pharmacologic therapy is recommended in patients with 10-year risk of major osteoporotic fracture of greater than 20% or hip fracture of 3%). Therefore, observation (c) is not appropriate. Estrogen (a) should be reserved for selected women with severe vasomotor symptoms, and usually within 5 years of menopause. Denosumab (d) and teriparatide (e) are not first-line therapies in most cases.

5. A 69-year-old male patient is admitted after being found on the street, lethargic and stuporous. Laboratory data shows serum calcium of 15.5 mg/dL (*N*: <11). His friend states that he is a heavy smoker and a chest X-ray demonstrates a large pulmonary mass. Which of the following supports a diagnosis of hypercalcemia from squamous cell carcinoma of the lung?
   a. Elevated serum PTH, low serum phosphate
   b. Elevated serum PTH-rP, high serum phosphate
   c. High serum osteoclast-activating factor, low serum phosphate
   d. High serumPTH-related peptide, low serum phosphate
   e. Elevated serum $1,25(OH)_2D$, low serum PTH-related peptide (PTH-rP) and PTH

   (d) This is a classic case of humoral hypercalcemia of malignancy (HHM) due to secretion of PTH-related peptide (PTH-rP), which has PTH-like actions and can result in hypophosphatemia (as with native PTH), although its effects on phosphate are not as pronounced as with PTH. (a) represents primary hyperparathyroidism, which is unlikely to present with severe acute hypercalcemia; PTH is suppressed in HHM. Osteoclast activating factors (OAFs) are seen in tumors producing localized osteolytic hypercalcemia (e.g., breast carcinoma).

6. A 57-year-old male presents to the emergency department with severe hypercalcemia, hyperphosphatemia, and acute renal failure. He has no medical problems except for type 2 diabetes treated with sitagliptin and hypertension treated with an angiotensin-converting enzyme (ACE) inhibitor. He is a non-smoker. Recently he has been having trouble with indigestion and has been taking an undisclosed number of antacids daily. His wife found a nearly empty bottle of flavored calcium carbonate tablets in his bedside stand. Serum PTH level is undetectable. Chest and abdominal CT scans done in the emergency department are normal. What is the most likely etiology of his illness?
   a. Primary hyperparathyroidism
   b. Hypercalcemia of malignancy
   c. Milk-alkali syndrome
   d. Sarcoidosis
   e. Side effect of DPP-IV inhibitor therapy

   (c) This is a classic case of milk-alkali syndrome due to overingestion of over-the-counter calcium supplements. Some people believe that if a small amount is good, a lot is better, and others think that "flavored" tablets are innocuous. This condition presents with hypercalcemia and renal failure, which leads to hyperphosphatemia.

7. A 47-year-old male patient presents with numerous vertebral fractures and has low bone mass assessed by dual photon absorptiometry. Which of the following would not be a cause of secondary osteoporosis?
   a. Ingestion of exogenous glucocorticoids
   b. Illicit use of testosterone cypionate
   c. Ingestion of exogenous thyroid hormone
   d. Panhypopituitarism
   e. Kallmann's syndrome

   (b) Abuse of testosterone can cause a variety of ills, but not osteoporosis; if anything, it will increase bone density.

Reproductive Endocrinology

REVIEW

Let us review what we learned in the last lecture. Calcium is an important ion in regulating many processes, including muscle contraction, transmission of impulses in the nervous system, and coagulation. It also is an important second messenger in hormone action. It is not under direct control by the pituitary gland or hypothalamus and is therefore not a "classic" endocrine hormone since it is not secreted by a gland.

Calcium is bound to serum proteins such as albumin. Only the free or unbound (ionized) portion of calcium is biologically active. The major source of calcium is the skeleton, which contains over 99% of the body's calcium stores. The main regulator of calcium metabolism is parathyroid hormone (PTH), which is made by the parathyroid glands. Parathyroid hormone secretion increases when hypocalcemia occurs.

Another hormone important in calcium metabolism is vitamin D. This may be obtained from the diet but also can be produced by exposing the skin to the sun. The hormone calcitonin is a weak antagonist to PTH, and has no biological significance in humans.

Hypercalcemia may be caused by several disorders. Mild hypercalcemia is most commonly caused by primary hyperparathyroidism and has few symptoms. The most effective treatment for hyperparathyroidism at this time is surgery, although the calcimimetic agent cinacalcet is effective in some patients (but is not a definitive solution to the problem). Severe hypercalcemia is often brought about by malignancy, and may cause neuromuscular suppression, psychosis, coma, and even death. Most commonly, malignancies produce hypercalcemia by secreting a substance called parathyroid hormone-related protein (PTH-rP). Other tumors may produce hypercalcemia by secreting factors that dissolve bone (osteoclast activating factors). Too much vitamin D can also cause hypercalcemia; this usually occurs when high-potency pharmacologic preparations are ingested. Milk-alkali syndrome results from the ingestion of excess alkaline substances (e.g., carbonate salts) and calcium, resulting in renal failure and metabolic alkalosis.

The treatment of hypercalcemia depends on the etiology. Primary hyperparathyroidism is normally treated by surgery. Care of malignancy-associated hypercalcemia includes treatment of the tumor and administration of antiresorptive agents, such as zoledronic acid and pamidronate.

Hypocalcemia causes neuromuscular excitability and may result in muscular spasms and seizures. One cause of hypercalcemia is hypoparathyroidism, in which the body produces too little parathyroid hormone. The treatment of hypoparathyroidism involves administration of potent vitamin D analogs such as calcitriol, since synthetic PTH is not widely available at this time for administration. Pseudohypoparathyroidism is another disorder that results from tissue resistance to PTH. These patients often have characteristic clinical features and have elevated PTH levels because of hormone resistance.

Bone is a rigid support for extremities, helps provide levers for locomotion and protection for vital organs, and also serves as a large reservoir for calcium and other ions. It is a living organism constantly being remodeled. Osteoporosis results when the amount of bone that is made is less than the amount that is resorbed. The most common cause of osteoporosis is hypogonadism in women, secondary to menopause or oophorectomy. Estrogen helps decrease the risk of osteoporosis but has many side effects; thus its administration is limited to specific individuals. Another common cause of osteoporosis is exposure to large amounts of glucocorticoids.

Osteoporosis is best diagnosed with a special X-ray study called DEXA. Treatments for osteoporosis include estrogen, calcium/vitamin D supplementation, bisphosphonates (e.g., alendronate), calcitonin, synthetic parathyroid hormone (teriparatide), RANKL inhibitors (denosumab), and estrogen-like drugs such as raloxifene.

AN INTRODUCTION TO REPRODUCTIVE ENDOCRINOLOGY

Reproduction is vital to the continued survival of any organism. In addition to propagation of the species, hormones secreted by the sex organs are important in other bodily processes. For example, sex steroids are necessary for normal bone metabolism. This lecture deals with the development and endocrine function of the reproductive systems in men and women.

In our football team analogy, think of the reproductive system as the scouts who look for new talent for the draft. If the team did not draft new players, the old players would retire and the team would cease to exist. The new players ensure that a vital core of players is present at all times.

REGULATION OF TESTICULAR FUNCTION

The testes contain two important cell types. Sertoli cells are the site of spermatogenesis, and are stimulated by the pituitary hormone follicle-stimulating hormone (FSH). The other cell of interest is the Leydig cell, the site of testosterone synthesis; the stimulus for this is luteinizing hormone (LH). As with most feedback loops, the trophic hormone (LH) is inhibited by the end product (testosterone) and high levels result in low LH levels. Other minor androgens (e.g., dehydroepiandrosterone, androstenedione) are also present, but testosterone is the major androgen of the reproductive system. A small proportion of testosterone in men originates in the adrenal cortex; in the normal adult man this is not significant.

The hypothalamic hormone GnRH (gonadotropin-hormone releasing hormone), when secreted in a pulsatile manner (every 60–90 min), stimulates gonadotropin (FSH and LH). But, if given continuously, GnRH actually results in paradoxical inhibition of gonadotropin secretion.

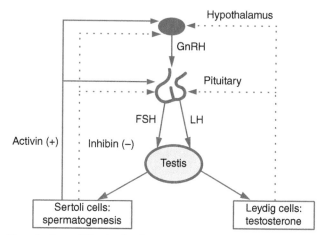

Regulation of Testicular Function

OVARIAN CYCLE REGULATION

The reproductive unit of the woman is the ovum, which contains theca and granulosa cells. Many follicles (groups of ova) develop in the ovary, but only one is destined to develop fully, and the others degenerate. The two main female sex steroids are estradiol and progesterone. Approximately 50% of testosterone in women originates in the ovaries, and the rest comes from the adrenal cortex and aromatization (conversion) of other steroids in peripheral tissues (e.g., fat). Estradiol is synthesized in several steps. Initially, androgenic precursors (testosterone and androstenedione) are made in the theca interna cells under the influence of luteinizing hormone (LH). The androgens are then aromatized to estradiol and estrone in the granulosa cells under the influence of FSH. This unique process is called the two-cell concept of ovarian steroid synthesis.

The ovarian cycle may be divided into follicular (proliferative) and luteal (secretory) phases. Like in the male, pulsatile secretion of hypothalamic GnRH facilitates secretion of the gonadotropins LH and FSH. Early in

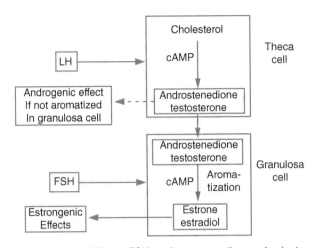

Two-Cell Concept of Ovarian Steroidogenesis

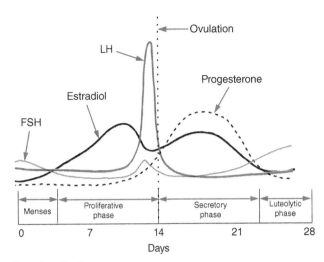

Ovarian Cycle

the follicular phase, FSH secretion predominates, which increases the number of follicles and granulosa cells. Only one of many follicles is destined to become "ripe" for ovulation. LH secretion then increases, leading to theca cell proliferation. As estradiol concentrations increase, FSH secretion decreases. During this phase, the endometrium thickens and grows in length, mucus is secreted from the cervix, and maturation of the vaginal epithelium occurs (due to the effects of estrogens). Most follicles regress as the FSH secretion diminishes, but hopefully one will have enough receptors to remain viable. This is the one selected to ovulate.

In the viable follicle, estradiol concentrations increase, and although estrogen normally inhibits LH production, in this instance there is a paradoxical switch from negative to positive feedback, resulting in a pituitary LH surge. This culminates in ovulation, and the ovum is expelled from the ovary.

Then, the granulosa cells also acquire LH receptors and begin to secrete progesterone (the luteal phase), with the formation of the corpus luteum. Progesterone concentrations continue to increase, the glands become longer and edematous, and estradiol levels remain high. If the ovum is not fertilized, involution of the corpus luteum (luteolysis) occurs, and the endometrium is sloughed away (menstruation).

If the ovum is fertilized, the fetoplacental unit begins secreting the glycoprotein hormone β-hCG (human chorionic gonadotropin). This maintains the hormonal secretion of the corpus luteum. (Pregnancy tests detect β-hCG in the blood or urine.) The elevated estrogen levels suppress FSH, preventing further ovulation.

GONADAL DIFFERENTIATION

The embryonic gonads are indistinguishable until about 6 weeks. If a Y chromosome is present (male), a special protein called testis-determining factor is secreted, and the embryonic gonad becomes a testis. If there is no Y chromosome (female), an ovary develops. This is the traditional "female by default" hypothesis.

The presence or absence of a testis also determines which internal structures develop. The functional Sertoli cells of the testis secrete a hormone called müllerian inhibitory factor (MIF), which causes the müllerian (female) structures (uterus, uterine tubes, cervix, and upper third of the vagina) to disappear. The wolffian (male) structures (epididymis, vas deferens, seminal vesicles, and ejaculatory ducts) then develop in this case. If there is no testis, MIF is not secreted and the müllerian structures develop while the wolffian structures become vestigial remnants.

The type of external genitalia also is determined by (you guessed it) the presence or absence of a functional testis. Up to about 8 weeks, the external genitalia may differentiate into those of either sex. A functional testis secretes small amounts of testosterone and causes the differentiation into male external genitalia. In the absence of a testis, female external genitalia develop.

EFFECTS OF SEX STEROIDS

Testosterone results in differentiation of the internal and external male genital system and growth of the

Gonadal differentiation

Embryonic gonad

Y chromosome present

Y chromosome absent

♂

♀

Müllerian inhibitory factory secreted

Uterus, uterine tubes, cervix, upper vagina involute

Wolffian structures develop

Müllerian inhibitory factory not secreted

Uterus, uterine tubes, cervix, upper vagina develop

Wolffian structures involute

Gonadal Differentiation

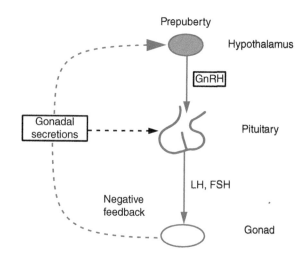

Low gonadal steroid levels result due to sensitivity of hypothalamus to very low circulating levels

Gonadal Axis in Childhood

scrotum, epididymis, vas deferens, seminal vesicles, prostate, and penis. It also results in skeletal muscle, laryngeal, and long bone growth in both sexes. Estradiol causes maturation of the vagina, uterus, and uterine tubes in women at puberty. It also alters the distribution and type of body fat to a more female or "gynecoid" type found on the hips, buttocks, and thighs. Typical male or "android" fat is more central (e.g., a beer belly) and predominantly in the abdomen.

Puberty

The newborn infant actually possesses all the "machinery" necessary to enter puberty and become sexually functional. Fortunately for the patient (and for society), this does not normally happen until the adolescent years (that's enough of a problem at that age!), because the hypothalamic–pituitary axis (HPA) is held in check by potent inhibitory mechanisms. In the prepubertal child, these very small circulating amounts of sex steroids inhibit gonadotropin secretion.

At puberty, the inhibition decreases, and the GnRH begins secreting in a pulsatile manner—every 60–90 min. This results in increased gonadotropin secretion and gonadal growth. The onset of gonadal development is termed gonadarche. The pulsatile secretion of GnRH is very important—if it is given continuously, LH and FSH secretion is paradoxically suppressed. Eventually, sex steroid levels remain at adult levels, where they remain throughout the reproductive years.

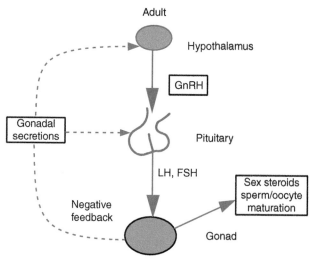

Adult levels of sex steroids and spermatocyte/ oocyte maturity occurs

Gonadal Axis in Adulthood

Ninety-nine percent of boys and girls will begin puberty between ages 9 and 14 and ages 8 and 13, respectively. Those who do not have onset of puberty by age 13 (F) or 14 (M) are said to have delayed puberty. Those with onset of puberty before age 8 (F) or 9 (M) are said to have precocious puberty.

Boys and girls start with relatively equal lean body mass. Due to the effects of testosterone, men end up on average with 1.5 times as much muscle mass and 0.5 times as much fat as women. There is, of course, individual variation, depending on genetics and environmental factors such as diet and exercise (some female athletes have more muscle mass and less fat than many men). Increased androgen secretion during puberty (men and women) results in deepening voice and acne. Sex steroids and growth hormone result in increased bone density, with peak values occurring in the mid-twenties. In both genders, testosterone increases muscle mass. In men, it increases bone density and spermatogenesis. Its effect on other tissues (external genitalia, prostate, and body hair) requires conversion by 5α-reductase to dihydrotestosterone (DHT).

Sex steroids result in an initial increase (spurt) in growth velocity, but eventually result in closing of the epiphyseal plates of long bones and cessation of growth. Since puberty begins earlier in girls than boys, the epiphyseal plates close sooner, resulting in women being shorter than men on average. Also, the effect of sex steroids on epiphyseal plates is primarily estradiol mediated, another reason that women are typically shorter. (Fusion of epiphyses in men occurs due to the extraglandular aromatization of testosterone to estradiol. Rarely, men with aromatase deficiency can continue to experience linear growth into their twenties.)

The Tanner stages refer to specific developmental milestones that occur in puberty. The stages are numbered 1 through 5: 1 is prepubertal, 5 is adult development, and 2–4 are in between. Girls typically start puberty sooner, with the initial sign of puberty in a girl being breast budding. The growth spurt starts earlier in girls, and ends sooner, for reasons described above. The first physical sign of puberty in a boy is testicular enlargement.

Adrenarche (also called pubarche) is another milestone of puberty and heralds the onset of adrenal androgen secretion. It is responsible for a large proportion of androgen secretion in girls. It is responsible for much of the terminal (dark, pigmented) hair in the axillary and pubic areas, and development of sweat glands in those areas (resulting in the characteristic pungent adult body odor). Terminal hair is coarse, pigmented, and has a greater potential for growth than vellus (fine, nonpigmented, "peach fuzz") hair. Terminal hair occurs on the scalp, eyebrows, and to varying degrees, on the body depending on the amount of circulating androgens and genetic differences in hair sensitivity. Vellus hair transforms into terminal hair given sufficient androgen

concentrations. This accounts for the typical heavy terminal hair growth (face, chest, and extremities) seen in men (although there is wide variation in men regarding the amount of hair). Pubic and axillary hair appears to require lower androgen concentrations than other hair for vellus to terminal transformation. The onset of puberty results in increased testosterone secretion and development of pubic and axillary hair and acne.

But, if testosterone causes terminal hair growth, why do many men (and occasional women) lose their head of hair as they age? Some terminal hairs, such as on the scalp, have a tendency to de-differentiate into miniaturized vellus hairs under the influence of testosterone and DHT. This is what happens in men with male pattern baldness (androgenetic alopecia). Not all men develop this; the susceptibility appears to be genetically transmitted (autosomal dominant) and is manifested as increased sensitivity of scalp hair to testosterone and DHT. Some women also develop androgenetic alopecia; it is not unique to men. 5α-reductase inhibitors such as finasteride can help reverse the "miniaturization" of follicles and restore hair growth in many patients.

Delayed puberty

Another common presenting complaint is delayed puberty. This is defined as the absence of any pubertal development in a boy of 14 or girl of 13. The most common cause is constitutional delay, in which the child is destined to develop normally but is simply delayed a few years. These persons do eventually go through puberty normally and reach a height appropriate for their genetic predispositions. There is often a positive family history in parents and older siblings. It is important to distinguish those with constitutional delay from those with organic disease (e.g., growth hormone deficiency). Growth charts in children with constitutional delay demonstrate early short stature, with eventual increase into the normal range. It is important to keep accurate height and weight records—it does not cost anything!

Another test, called a bone age (BA) study, is also useful. This simple test compares an X-ray of the wrist bones to a set of normal X-rays. Bones characteristically change with age, until the epiphyses fuse. Normally, bone age (BA) equals chronologic age (CA) during the developmental years. In those with delayed puberty, the full effect of sex steroids has not been realized, and the bone age is delayed (BA < CA). Children with early onset (precocious) puberty have BA > CA. BA therefore can be used to estimate a child's remaining growth.

Pathological causes of delayed puberty include hypopituitarism (due to growth hormone and/or gonadotropin deficiency), hypothyroidism, hypogonadism, and chromosomal abnormalities.

Precocious puberty

Precocious puberty (PP) is defined as the onset of secondary sexual development in a girl before age 8 or a boy before age 9. Most commonly, PP is central (complete or "true"), meaning that puberty occurs via premature activation of the HPA. It is called true because it occurs by the same mechanism as normal puberty, except at an earlier age. Peripheral ("incomplete") PP is caused by abnormal gonadotropin and/or sex steroid secretion, rather than premature activation of the HPA.

As we discussed earlier, the potential for pubertal development is present at birth, but is held in check by strong inhibitory mechanisms. If these are disturbed, puberty commences and sexual maturation and fertility are achieved. Any central nervous system lesion that disrupts the normal inhibitory responses can cause this (e.g., hydrocephalus and central nervous system tumors). Central PP may also be "idiopathic," where no obvious cause may be found.

Incomplete or peripheral PP may be caused by any condition that results in increased gonadotropin and/or sex steroid secretion (exogenous steroids, premature adrenarche, congenital adrenal hyperplasia, steroid-secreting adrenal tumors, steroid-secreting ovarian/testicular tumors, and gonadotropin-secreting tumors).

In all forms of PP, since sex steroid secretion occurs at an early age, premature skeletal growth and epiphyseal closure occurs, resulting in early tall stature but eventual short stature (which is irreversible). Early sexual development may also be psychologically devastating to the child, for obvious reasons.

Just like constitutional delayed puberty, a child may have constitutional early puberty. There is typically a family history of such and these children are often overweight. These children are large for their age but stop growing early at a normal adult height. As seen here, the growth curve appears normal but is shifted to the left by 2 or 3 years (the opposite of constitutional delay).

The treatment for central PP is to somehow "shut off" the HPA. Nature has, fortunately, provided us an elegant way to accomplish this; administration of long-acting GnRH analogs such as leuprolide cause paradoxical gonadotropin suppression when given continuously (remember that GnRH only stimulates the pituitary when secreted in pulsatile manner). The child is given these drugs until the agent is withdrawn at the appropriate age, and the child goes through puberty normally.

Treatment for peripheral PP involves locating the site of steroid excess (e.g., tumor, congenital adrenal enzyme defect) and treating it (e.g., surgical removal, medical therapy).

Hypogonadism

Hypogonadism is the condition of sex steroid deficiency. It may be primary (due to a gonadal defect). This is also termed hypergonadotropic hypogonadism because gonadotropin levels (from the pituitary gland) are elevated. Secondary (lack of gonadotropin secretion) or tertiary (lack of GnRH) forms of hypogonadism are called hypogonadotropic hypogonadism.

A famous drawing by Leonardo de Vinci depicted a man with his hands stretched out and fitting perfectly into a square box; even then, this brilliant man realized these "ideal" human proportions. In a normal person, therefore, arm span roughly equals height, and the ratio of the upper to the lower body segment is approximately one.

In hypogonadal states, however, body proportions become abnormal. Sex steroids initially cause an acceleration of bone age during the growth spurt. Although all long bones have a finite potential for growth, sex steroids (mainly estradiol, in both genders) eventually hasten closure of the epiphyses and cessation of linear growth (testosterone is aromatized to estradiol in men, producing this effect). Sex steroid secretion peaks a bit earlier in girls than in boys, resulting in girls being initially taller than boys (due to earlier onset of puberty and predominant effect of estradiol) and stopping growth sooner (because of earlier epiphyseal fusion). With inadequate sex steroid secretion, bone age may be delayed a bit. However, they do continue to grow under the influence of growth hormone, and because of the lack of effect on epiphyseal closure, the long bones grow longer than they should, leading to disproportionately long arms and legs. This person no longer fits inside the square, as the arms are too long. The lower body segment is also longer than the upper body segment. These abnormalities are termed hypogonadal or eunuchoidal body proportions.

In an adult with hypogonadism, measuring body proportions is one way to tell whether the problem began prior to or after puberty; if the proportions are normal, the defect occurred in adulthood, after normal growth had ceased.

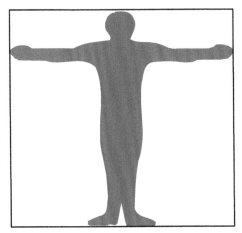

Normal body proportions
Arm span = height
Upper = lower body segment

Normal Body Proportions

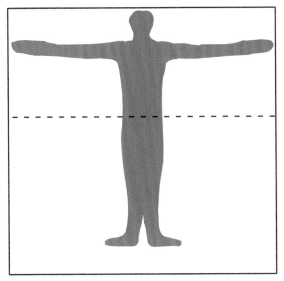

Hypogonadal or eunuchoidal proportions
Arm span > height
Upper < lower body segment

Hypogonadal (Eunuchoidal) Body Proportions

We all know that all women in middle age go through an abrupt decline in ovarian function called the menopause. Some have proposed a similar phenomenon in men, called the "andropause," in which male hormone levels abruptly decline, but there is little evidence to suggest any such phenomenon. Most men retain sexual function and fertility well into the sixth and seventh decades of life (the risk for genetic mutations increases with advanced paternal age, although not to the extent of women who conceive in the latter stages of their reproductive cycle). Testosterone levels decline approximately 1–2% each year after age 30.

Before a diagnosis of hypogonadism can be considered, the practitioner must be certain that testosterone deficiency truly exists. A common error is measuring testosterone in the afternoon; in fact, this is when levels are the lowest. This may be a biologically programmed throwback to our "hunter-gatherer" days, where the most difficult work (fighting and looking for food) took place early in the day; in fact, many human hormones (cortisol, growth hormone, testosterone) are highest then. Therefore, testosterone levels should be measured in the morning.

Also remember from the first lecture that sex steroids are protein bound (to a molecule called sex-hormone binding globulin (SHBG)). There are several conditions that can alter the SHBG level (thereby changing the total level). The most common condition is obesity, which can lower SHBG and total testosterone levels; here, measuring free testosterone and SHBG levels is often indicated.

Hypogonadotropic hypogonadism

This type of hypogonadism (a secondary deficiency) is caused by a defect in either GnRH (hypothalamus) or gonadotropin (LH and FSH) secretion. The most common cause is Kallmann syndrome, a disorder of GnRH secretion associated with anosmia (inability to smell). Other midline defects, such as a cleft palate or unilateral renal agenesis, may be seen. It is seen much more often in men and is due most commonly to a defect in the KAL-1 gene (on the X chromosome) or FGFR1 (autosomal dominant), which code for a protein called anosmin. PROKR2 and PROK2 mutations also cause the disorder. The interesting thing about Kallmann syndrome is that patients do not realize they cannot smell until you test them, because they do not understand the concept of "smell"—it is like asking a congenitally blind person to describe color; there is no perspective. Sense of smell can be qualitatively measured with any number of things commonly available at a supermarket: coffee, garlic, wintergreen, fruit extract, and so on. More sophisticated methods of testing smell (using a device called an olfactometer) are available but rarely necessary.

Hypogonadotropic hypogonadism may also be caused by any condition that disrupts pituitary function (e.g., hypopituitarism, hypothalamic destruction).

The treatment of hypogonadotropic hypogonadism depends on the desired result. If fertility is not desired, testosterone (male) or estrogen (female) replacement is given. If fertility is desired, gonadal stimulation can be induced by administration of gonadotropins. The glycoprotein β-hCG has LH-like activity and is given along with FSH. Fertility can be induced in both sexes, but is more difficult in women because of the greater complexity of the female reproductive cycle. Alternatively, GnRH may be given in pulsatile manner by a subcutaneous infusion pump, which induces LH and FSH secretion by the pituitary. It must be given in pulses every 90 min, since continuous therapy results in paradoxical suppression of the pituitary.

Hypergonadotropic hypogonadism

Hypergonadotropic hypogonadism is due to a primary gonadal defect, and results in high gonadotropin levels (since the hypothalamus and pituitary function normally). In men, the most common cause is a chromosomal abnormality called Klinefelter syndrome, occurring in 1 in 1,000 men. In women, the most common cause is Turner syndrome, with an incidence of 1 in 2,500 girls). Other causes are less common and include congenital anorchia, cryptorchidism, gonadal damage (chemotherapy, radiation therapy), gonadectomy, and mumps orchitis.

Men with Klinefelter syndrome typically have a 47, XXY cell karyotype (46, XY is normal). Testes are usually small and hard, and do not function properly. Since testosterone levels are deficient during adolescence, "eunuchoidal" proportions develop. Gynecomastia (male breast enlargement) is common, and these individuals have a higher incidence of breast carcinoma and other problems (e.g., mediastinal germ cell tumors). Intelligence is normal. Patients are generally infertile.

Turner syndrome is the most common cause of primary amenorrhea in girls and is associated with the absence of an X chromosome (45, X). Intelligence is normal. While many children with hypogonadism have relatively tall stature (due to delayed epiphyseal fusion), girls with Turner syndrome have short stature, due to a mutation in the short stature homeobox (SHOX) gene on the X chromosome; this condition often responds to growth hormone therapy, even though GH secretion is normal.

The characteristic physical abnormalities may include short stature, webbed neck, congenital heart or kidney abnormalities, coarctation of the aorta, cubitus valgus, and other associated endocrine diseases (e.g., hypothyroidism, diabetes mellitus, and many autoimmune diseases).

Treatment of hypergonadotropic hypogonadism consists of giving replacement steroids (estrogen or testosterone). Fertility is not possible, as spermatogenesis or oogenesis is absent or defective. Women with Turner

syndrome can have a viable pregnancy with an egg donor (fertilized *in vitro* with the partner's sperm); the fertilized ovum can then be implanted into the woman's uterus; the fetoplacental unit (an independent endocrine organ) can then develop normally and progress as a normal pregnancy.

Signs and Symptoms of Testosterone Deficiency in Men

Children	Adults
Decreased sexual maturation	Depression
Delayed puberty	Loss of energy
Short stature (if associated with other hormonal deficiencies)	Loss of libido
Eunuchoidal (hypogonadal) proportions	Diminished muscle mass
	Erectile dysfunction

Testosterone replacement

Testosterone is well absorbed by the intestine, but is virtually useless because it is rapidly degraded in the liver by something called the first-pass effect. Testosterone may be combined with an ester, producing a long-lasting compound that may be given intramuscularly. These testosterone esters are generally given every 2 weeks to 1 month. Transdermal testosterone is available, and is administered as a once-daily patch or gel preparation, applied to the skin once daily. Oral derivatives of testosterone that resist hepatic degradation are available; however, these compounds have been shown to cause liver damage and their use is not recommended for treatment of hypogonadism.

Androgens carry a high potential for abuse and unfortunately have been used by some strength athletes, sometimes in doses 100–1,000 times normal. Abuse of these drugs causes a variety of psychological and physiological problems, and illicit use of androgens is illegal in the United States and many other countries and banned by all amateur and professional sports organizations.

A final problem is that direct-to-consumer advertising has created the impression that male hypogonadism is a very common problem and that restoration of levels will work miracles. True hypogonadism is not ubiquitous, and, while therapy of a truly hypogonadal man will create beneficial metabolic effects, one must be realistic about the potential benefits.

In addition, testosterone therapy is not like taking a vitamin or energy drink. It is a hormone with potent metabolic effects. Not all of these effects are beneficial. As mentioned earlier, the most important issue is to make certain that the diagnosis is correct to begin with (e.g., do not base a diagnosis on a late-afternoon testosterone level, when readings are lowest). Testosterone may worsen prostatic hyperplasia, creating difficulties with urination. Testosterone stimulates erythrocyte production and may produce erythrocytosis (increase in hematocrit), which can have deleterious effects. Finally, testosterone may cause or worsen obstructive sleep apnea in susceptible individuals (e.g., obese men). Therefore, it is not a therapy to be begun haphazardly.

Finally, the diagnosis of male hypogonadism must be made properly. Testosterone is secreted in cyclical manner, with the highest levels in the morning; consequently, measuring levels in the late afternoon lead to misleading results, as levels are at a physiologic low then. The level should be measured in the morning, with free (unbound) levels being measured in patients who likely have SHBG abnormalities (e.g., obese patients).

Estrogen replacement

Like testosterone, estradiol is well absorbed orally but rapidly degraded by the first pass phenomenon. Micronized estradiol, however, produces satisfactory plasma levels. Conjugated estrogens have high bioavailability and are prepared from the urine of pregnant mares. Other compounds include esterified estrogens, estropipate, and ethinyl estradiol.

Estrogen was once widely prescribed to all menopausal women, but multiple studies have demonstrated hazards (most notably an increase in the risk of cardiovascular and thromboembolic disease) in women taking estrogen. Therefore, candidates for estrogen therapy should be selected very carefully and estrogen used only for certain indications (e.g., disabling vasomotor symptoms—and then only for a brief period of time (5 years or less)). Alternative therapies for vasomotor symptoms (e.g., selective serotonin uptake inhibitors) are available, with varying degrees of efficacy.

Estrogen therapy in women of premenopausal age is a different matter. Women with premature ovarian failure (before age 40), Turner syndrome, and so on, should be given estrogen, as this promotes normal bone health. The exception would be in those individuals with contraindications (e.g., breast cancer).

Women without a uterus may take continuous estrogen alone. Synthetic progestin (medroxyprogesterone) should be given to women who still have a uterus. One method is administering the estrogen for the first part of the month and adding progestin to the last week of the month, with withdrawal of both drugs for several days. This results in withdrawal menses similar to that of natural menses. This ensures that the uterine lining is sloughed each month, since unopposed estrogen stimulation leads to endometrial buildup, which can result in endometrial carcinoma. Another method is administering the estrogen and progestin continuously. This also decreases endometrial buildup and results in less bleeding than treatment with intermittent therapy.

Estrogen can also be given transdermally. The lipid-lowering effect is less when administered transdermally, since less estrogen passes through the liver (the site of lipoprotein synthesis). Those with a uterus are also given continuous progestin.

In addition to the risks mentioned above, estrogen should not be given to women with a history of breast cancer, as estradiol may stimulate tumor growth. Estrogen administration also results in a very small increase in breast cancer in all women, so women with a strong family history should probably not take it, although this is not an absolute contraindication. Estrogen should be avoided in those with active thromboembolic disease (e.g., recent pulmonary embolism on anticoagulant therapy) or those with the common Leiden factor V mutation (resistance to activated protein C), which predisposes patients to thromboembolism.

Selective estrogen receptor modulators (SERMs), such as raloxifene, appear to have protective effects against osteoporosis. These drugs do not help with vasomotor flashes, however. Like estrogen, they appear to increase the incidence of thromboembolism in susceptible individuals.

Gynecomastia

Gynecomastia is the presence of abnormal breast enlargement in men. It may occur whenever there is a decrease in the androgen:estrogen (A:E) ratio. This may happen with either androgen deficiency or estrogen excess. The most common cause is pubertal gynecomastia. Early in puberty, testicular steroidogenesis favors estrogen secretion. As puberty progresses, steroid synthesis favors androgen production, and pubertal gynecomastia disappears in most cases.

Obese boys also tend to have higher estrogen levels due to the peripheral conversion of androgen to estrogen in fat; incidence of gynecomastia in them is higher. One must distinguish lipomastia (increased fat in the breast area) from true gynecomastia, since often the large breast appearance is simply fat.

Hypogonadism may obviously cause gynecomastia by decreasing the A:E ratio. It is very common in Klinefelter syndrome. Adults may develop gynecomastia if hypogonadism occurs (e.g., men undergoing orchiectomy for prostate cancer). Many commonly used medications interfere with androgen production and may cause gynecomastia. Finally, marijuana contains biologically active phytoestrogens and its use may produce gynecomastia—just one more reason to tell patients not to use it!

Steroid-producing (adrenal, testis) or β-hCG-producing (testis, lung) neoplasms can cause gynecomastia. Acromegaly results in soft tissue growth and can be another cause. It may also be associated with hypogonadism and/or hyperprolactinemia.

Pubertal gynecomastia is typically self-limited, and underlying disorders (e.g., hypogonadism, germ cell tumors) should be treated. In severe cases, a reduction mammoplasty should be considered. Patients with Klinefelter syndrome have a higher incidence of breast carcinoma and should be checked regularly.

Primary amenorrhea

Amenorrhea is the absence of menses. It is classified as primary (menses have never occurred) or secondary (menses have occurred before but have now stopped).

The most common cause of primary amenorrhea is Turner syndrome. Classic Turner syndrome (45, XO gonadal dysgenesis) is fairly common (1 in 2,500 live female births) and results in primordial, nonfunctional ovaries. This disorder has already been discussed in some detail.

Müllerian agenesis is another common cause of primary amenorrhea. As the name implies, it is associated with absent müllerian structures. Since there is no uterus, menses cannot occur. The ovaries are normal and hence secondary sex characteristics are normal. Testicular feminization (discussed below) is the third most common cause of primary amenorrhea.

Secondary amenorrhea

Secondary amenorrhea is a condition in which menses have occurred previously but have stopped. In young women, the most common cause is anovulation. Polycystic ovary syndrome (PCOS), to be discussed in detail later, is a common cause of anovulation in reproductive-age women. In older women, primary

ovarian failure (menopause) is most likely. Other causes include hypothalamic amenorrhea, hypopituitarism, and hyperprolactinemia. Uterine outflow tract obstruction may cause secondary amenorrhea. In this case, the ovaries function normally, but menses cannot occur since menstrual outflow is blocked.

Evaluation of amenorrhea

The first goal is to determine if the ovaries are producing estrogen. Although estradiol levels can be measured, a simpler, dynamic method of determining adequate estrogenization is a progestin challenge. In this test, a synthetic progesterone derivative (medroxyprogesterone) is given for several days. If adequate estrogenization has occurred, the menstrual lining (which has been "primed" by estrogen) will be sloughed off several days after administration of progestin. If withdrawal bleeding occurs after the progestin has been given for several days, this confirms adequate estrogenization and means that the amenorrhea is due to inadequate progesterone secretion (anovulation). If there is no withdrawal bleeding after progestin, a combination of estrogen and progestin is given. If withdrawal bleeding occurs, it suggests inadequate estrogenization (e.g., ovarian failure, hypothalamic amenorrhea). If there is no bleeding with combination therapy, there is either a mechanical outflow obstruction or no uterus present.

Hypothalamic amenorrhea is a functional abnormality in GnRH secretion resulting in low gonadotropin levels and secondary amenorrhea. It is common in young women with increased psychological stress (e.g., going away to college, breaking up with a partner, starting a new job). It typically is a self-limited disorder. Eating disorders such as anorexia nervosa can result in hypothalamic amenorrhea as well as other serious health issues. Other causes of hypogonadotropic amenorrhea include hypopituitarism and hyperprolactinemia.

Consequences of estrogen deficiency in women

Early estrogen deficiency leads to vaginal atrophy and dyspareunia (painful intercourse). A decrease in estrogen levels leads to stimulation of central thermoregulatory centers, with resultant vasomotor or hot flashes. The mechanism is unknown. Women who have a sudden decrease in estrogen (e.g., after oophorectomy) experience hot flashes to a greater degree than those with a slower decrease (e.g., natural menopause).

In the long term, estrogen deficiency may cause decreased bone mass and osteoporosis. This is a "high-turnover" form of osteoporosis, and most of the bone is lost within the first 10–15 years after menopause. It is therefore most beneficial to replace estrogen as soon as possible after menopause.

Estrogen in post-menopausal women was once felt to have beneficial cardiovascular effects, including increase in HDL cholesterol and decrease in LDL cholesterol. Estrogen deficiency leads to increase in android (central) obesity, which is more atherogenic than gynecoid obesity. However, as mentioned above, we also know that estrogen therapy leads to increased cardiovascular disease and thromboembolic events despite biochemical improvements in the lipid profile. Estrogen should be reserved for selected women with low risk for cardiovascular disease (e.g., women with disabling vasomotor flashes). Even then, therapy should be continued for the shortest time possible (e.g., 5 years or less).

Hirsutism

Hirsutism refers to the condition of excess terminal (pigmented) hair in women. Let us review the physiology of hair growth. Vellus hair is "miniaturized" hair that is soft, fine, and nonpigmented, and transforms into terminal (coarse, pigmented) hair after stimulation by androgen. Terminal hair is androgen dependent, except on the scalp and eyebrows. In these areas, androgens have the opposite effect. In many men, the terminal hair on the scalp is sensitive to androgen, causing reverse transformation to vellus hair (androgenetic alopecia, male pattern baldness, discussed earlier). Androgenetic alopecia may occur in women if androgen levels and/or hair sensitivity to androgen (due to genetically determined factors) is high enough.

Women normally have terminal hair only on the scalp, eyebrows, and "adrenarchal" areas (axilla, pubic area). There is a marked genetic difference in the amount of terminal hair expressed due to variability in androgen sensitivity; androgen levels are similar among all ethnic groups. The goal is to rule out serious underlying disease.

One must distinguish hirsutism (the presence of excess terminal hair) from virilization (development of other masculine qualities such as increased muscle mass, deepening of the voice, and baldness). Virilization is much more suggestive of endocrine disease than simple hirsutism.

Most cases of hirsutism result from increased sensitivity to normal amounts of androgen (familial or idiopathic hirsutism). Some ethnic groups simply manifest more body hair than others, although actual androgen levels are similar. Any endocrine disorder resulting in an increased androgen-to-estrogen ratio may cause hirsutism, including virilizing adrenal and/or ovarian tumors, congenital adrenal hyperplasia, and PCOS.

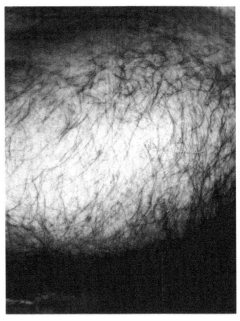

Severe Hirsutism Secondary to Virilizing Ovarian Tumor

The treatment of hirsutism includes treatment of underlying disorders, if present. Many drugs are useful in the treatment of hirsutism. One class of drugs, the antiandrogens, blocks the effect of testosterone on its receptor; the most commonly used is the aldosterone antagonist/diuretic spironolactone (the newer agent eplerenone does not have this effect). Oral contraceptives decrease the androgen to estrogen ratio by increasing estrogen levels. DHT production is held back by 5α-reductase inhibitors (e.g., finasteride), with reduction in terminal hair. All these drugs can have adverse effects on a fetus; therefore, be certain that the woman is not pregnant. A topical drug, eflornithine, inhibits ornithine decarboxylase, an enzyme necessary for hair follicle development.

Cosmetic treatments for hirsutism include simply shaving or bleaching the hair. Removal of hair (epilation) can be accomplished by several methods. Electrolysis utilizes an electric current that permanently destroys the hair follicle, and many treatments may be required. Laser epilation has also shown promise as a treatment for hirsutism. Waxing, although commonly employed in this country, may actually cause increased irritation and worsen the problem if used repeatedly.

Polycystic ovary syndrome (PCOS)

PCOS is a common disorder of chronic anovulation leading to increased estrogen production and infertility. To understand this disorder, remember the two-cell concept of steroidogenesis we discussed earlier. LH (luteinizing hormone) primarily stimulates the theca cells, which synthesize androgen from cholesterol. Androgens, in turn, are aromatized to estrogen in the granulosa cells under the influence of FSH.

Women with PCO are sort of stuck in a "time warp" at the middle of the reproductive cycle—their ovaries are trying desperately to ovulate in order to try and break the vicious cycle. Without ovulation, FSH levels are lower and androgen secretion predominates as a result. Instead, the increased LH levels lead to even more androgen production. Until this cycle is broken, the problem continues.

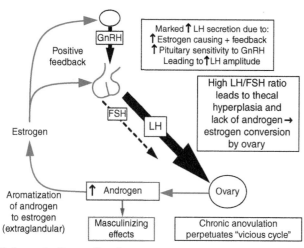

Polycystic Ovary Syndrome

The characteristic woman with PCOS has chronic anovulation, "android" obesity, hyperinsulinism, and hyperandrogenism. These components occur in varying degrees: not all women are obese, for example. Some have only minimal hirsutism, whereas in many it is quite severe.

Android obesity often results in hyperinsulinemia (insulin resistance) due to defective insulin receptor action and may lead to glucose intolerance and type 2 diabetes mellitus. Hyperinsulinemia, in turn, may increase androgen production, worsening the problem. Hyperandrogenism may then impair insulin action, leading to another vicious cycle.

Android fat is also metabolically active in aromatizing estrogen to androgen, and thus obesity also plays a role.

Hyperandrogenism itself can impair insulin action, which perpetuates the vicious cycle so predominant in PCOS.

The treatment of PCOS depends on the desired result. If the woman wants to have children, ovulation must be induced. This is typically performed with the estrogen agonist clomiphene citrate. This compound effectively inhibits the effects of stronger estrogens and permits gonadotropins to be secreted normally, allowing for ovulation. Other agents such as FSH may be used if this fails. Insulin-sensitizing drugs such as metformin and the thiazolidinediones (TZDs) theoretically improve symptoms by decreasing insulin resistance. They have been used in patients with severe insulin resistance who have not responded to other therapies.

If fertility is not desired, a progestin may simply be given at the end of the month to induce withdrawal bleeding. This is necessary because the endometrium is hyperplastic and is at higher risk for transforming into endometrial carcinoma if not sloughed regularly. Hirsutism may be treated with the methods above. Weight loss may decrease hyperinsulinism and improve symptoms in obese women.

Disorders of sexual differentiation (DSD)

Hermaphroditos, a character of ancient Greek mythology, was the son of Hermes and Aphrodite. The gods joined his body with that of a nymph who loved him, forming a single being who was both male and female—Hermaphrodite. The term hermaphrodism has persisted and has been applied to many intersex conditions, but true hermaphrodism (ovotesticular disorder of sexual differentiation (DSD)) is an extremely rare condition in which both ovarian and testicular tissues are found in the same individual. Pseudohermaphroditism is a more common condition in which the phenotype (appearance) is opposite to that of the genetic sex; for example, a female pseudohermaphrodite has a 46, XX (female) karyotype but appears male. A male pseudohermaphrodite appears female but has a 46, XY (male) karyotype. The most common cause in women is the 21α-hydroxylase variant of congenital adrenal hyperplasia, which we discussed in Lecture 4. Causes in males include the feminizing forms of congenital adrenal hyperplasia and testicular feminization.

Recently, the term "disorders of sexual differentiation (DSD)" has been recommended to replace the terms "pseudohermaphrodite," "hermaphrodite," and "intersex," which are confusing and even pejorative.

The differentiation of external and internal genitalia is highly variable, and most often ambiguous external genitalia are present in patients with DSDs. One exception is testicular feminization: a relatively common cause of primary amenorrhea and 46, XY DSD (older term: male pseudohermaphrodism) in girls. These women are in fact genotypic males (46, XY) who lack testosterone receptors, resulting in end-organ insensitivity to androgen, resulting in a hormone resistance syndrome. Since testosterone has no effect, wolffian (male) structures are absent, and müllerian (female) structures (uterus, uterine tubes, upper vagina) are absent, since the testes make MIF. In the complete form, total lack of masculinization occurs, leading to a normal female phenotype; indeed, in the typical case, no endocrine disorder is suspected until primary amenorrhea is discovered. A female hurdler with complete testicular feminization was in fact disqualified many years ago from the Olympics because of a 46, XY karyotype, despite the fact that she appeared to be a normal woman and the disorder confers no competitive advantage over other women. Girls with complete testicular feminization have only vellus hairs (except on the scalp and eyebrows, which do not depend on androgen for transformation to terminal hair). Because of decreased androgen effect, they often do not suffer from acne to the extent of their teenage peers, and their voices may be higher pitched than other girls. They can lead normal lives as women (except for the inability to reproduce, of course).

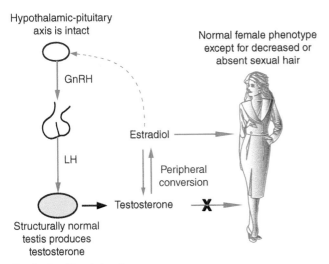

Testicular Feminization

You may wonder how adequate estrogen is produced since these individuals lack ovaries. Testosterone of testicular origin is aromatized to estradiol in the peripheral compartment (i.e., fat). Levels are thus in the normal female range.

These girls have a normal female appearance and therefore are raised as such. They should always be referred to as female since this is their phenotypic appearance, and no reference should be made to their genetic karyotype. To tell these girls that they are really male is inappropriate, serves no logical purpose, and may cause significant psychological problems.

The undescended (cryptorchid) testes are at higher risk for malignancy and should be removed at adulthood. Supplemental estrogen must then be given until the average age of menopause, as the source of estrogen will be gone (estrogen deficiency in reproductive age women can result in health problems such as osteoporosis). Since there is no uterus, menses obviously cannot occur, so a progestin is unnecessary. Only the lower portion of the vagina is present, and ends in a blind pouch. Usually, a vagina long enough to permit intercourse is achievable by slowly introducing larger forms to stretch it. In some cases, reconstructive surgery may be required.

Another, less common form of 46, XY DSD is 5α-reductase deficiency. While testosterone itself has direct effects on many tissues during male puberty (increasing muscle mass, voice deepening, growth spurt, etc.), the external genitalia and hair follicles require conversion of testosterone to DHT.

In this disorder, the genitalia are female or ambiguous due to the failure of conversion of testosterone to DHT. If recognized early, DHT can be topically applied to the genital area, resulting in substantial growth (although some corrective surgery may still be required). If not recognized, then a serious problem results if the child is reared as female. At the time of pubarche, testosterone levels increase, resulting in appearance of male secondary sexual characteristics (except for diminished facial hair growth and genital development). This "female to male" transformation at puberty can be perplexing to clinicians in societies lacking specialty medical care.

REVIEW QUESTIONS

1. A 17-year-old man presents with gynecomastia and decreased sexual maturation. Examination reveals a tall man (height 72 in. (183 cm)) with arm span greater than height; he has moderate bilateral gynecomastia with small testes measuring 5 mL in volume each (normal 25 mL). Serum AM testosterone is very low, and serum FSH/LH levels are several times elevated. Thyroid profile and other routine serum chemistries are normal. The most likely diagnosis is:
   a. Kallmann syndrome
   b. Klinefelter syndrome
   c. Hypopituitarism
   d. Mumps orchitis

   (b) This is a classic presentation of Klinefelter syndrome, with hypogonadal proportions, gynecomastia, small testes, and elevated gonadotropins (which would be low in Kallmann syndrome (a)). Hypopituitarism (c) would likely result in short stature. Mumps is unlikely given that all children are vaccinated; even so, it does not result in hypogonadism in children.

2. A 16-year-old girl presents with primary amenorrhea. She developed normally and does well in school and athletics. She is 69 in. (175 cm) tall and weighs 141 lb (64 kg). She has normal female secondary sex characteristics, and examination is normal except for the absence of terminal hair in the axillary and pubic area. You are unable to palpate ovaries or a uterus; vagina ends in a blind pouch with no cervix visible. The most likely etiology is:
   a. Turner syndrome
   b. Hypopituitarism
   c. Congenital adrenal hyperplasia
   d. Androgen resistance syndrome (testicular feminization)
   e. Uterine outflow tract obstruction

   (d) This is a classic presentation of complete androgen resistance or testicular feminization syndrome, a 46, XY DSD (disorder of sexual differentiation). Keys to the diagnosis are a normal female habitus, absence of uterus/ovaries, and lack of terminal hair (except on the scalp and eyebrows). Girls with Turner syndrome (a) usually have short stature and lack of normal sexual development; same with hypopituitarism (b). There are feminizing forms of congenital adrenal hyperplasia (c), but they do not result in a completely normal female appearance. Uterine outflow tract obstruction (e) in a girl this age (imperforate hymen) would be readily diagnosed by pelvic examination.

Lipid Disorders

REVIEW

In the last lecture we learned about the function of the reproductive system. The testes contain two major cell types. The first are the Sertoli cells (the site of spermatogenesis), which are under the influence of follicle-stimulating hormone; they are the site of spermatogenesis. The Leydig cells are under the influence of luteinizing hormone and secrete testosterone. Under the pulsatile secretion of the hypothalamic hormone GnRH, the pituitary produces appropriate levels of FSH and LH. If GnRH is given continuously, however, a paradoxical decrease in gonadotropin secretion occurs.

Control of the ovary is more complex. The female reproductive unit is the ovum, which contains both theca and granulosa cells. Many follicles develop in the ovary during each cycle, but only one is destined to develop fully.

The ovarian cycle is divided into follicular and luteal phases. In the follicular phase, estradiol concentrations increase after a pituitary LH surge results in ovulation. In the luteal phase, the corpus luteum is formed with increasing progesterone secretion. If fertilization does not occur, the corpus luteum involutes, resulting in the loss of the endometrium during menstruation. If fertilization does occur, the fetoplacental unit begins secreting β-hCG to help maintain the hormonal environment of the corpus luteum, necessary for pregnancy.

The major female sex steroids are estradiol and progesterone. Much of the androgen in women also originates in the ovaries, and the rest comes from the adrenal cortex and other endogenous sources (aromatization in the periphery (fat)). Androgens are primarily made in the theca cells, whereas estrogens are produced by the granulosa cells (the "two-cell" concept of ovarian steroidogenesis).

The embryonic gonads are indistinguishable until about 6 weeks. If a Y chromosome is present, the embryonic gonad becomes a testis; if there is no Y chromosome, the gonad becomes an ovary. The same occurs with the internal structures and external genitalia. If a testis is present, internal male structures and external male genitalia develop. In the absence of a testis, female internal structures and female external genitalia develop. This is the traditional "female by default" hypothesis.

Puberty is a complex process that involves the hypothalamic–pituitary axis. All the mechanisms necessary for going to puberty are present at birth and are held in check by strong inhibitory mechanisms. Girls tend to start puberty earlier than boys; 99% of girls and boys begin the process of puberty by ages 13 and 14, respectively. The adrenal glands also secrete testosterone and are important in puberty; this hormonal event is called adrenarche.

Most of the time, delayed puberty is not pathological and is simply a variation of normal (called constitutional delay of puberty). X-rays of the wrist can be compared with normal standards to assess skeletal maturation; this is called a bone age study and is useful to assess the potential for further growth; delayed bone age means that more potential linear growth remains. Pathological endocrine causes of delayed puberty include hypopituitarism and hypogonadism.

Precocious puberty is the opposite of delayed puberty and, like the latter, is often just a variation from normal. Pathological precocious puberty results in eventual short adult stature because of premature fusion of the epiphyseal plates caused by early exposure of the skeleton to excess sex steroids.

Hypogonadism may be primary or secondary. Persons who develop hypogonadism before complete skeletal maturation develop what is called hypogonadal (eunuchoidal) proportions in which the arms and legs are disproportionately long due to lack of the sex steroid effect (primarily estradiol) on epiphyseal fusion. Conversely, hypogonadism that begins after complete skeletal maturation does not alter the skeletal proportions.

Hypogonadism resulting from decreased gonadotropin levels is called hypogonadotropic hypogonadism and is the result of primary gonadal failure. Klinefelter syndrome is the most common cause of hypergonadotropic hypogonadism in males. Turner syndrome is another common cause of hypergonadotropic hypogonadism that occurs in females. Hypogonadism is easily treated with testosterone and estrogen supplementation, which restores secondary sex characteristics (but generally not fertility).

Amenorrhea (the absence of menses) is a common complaint in women. Females with primary amenorrhea have never had a menstrual period; those with secondary amenorrhea have had menses previously, but they have stopped. The most common cause of primary amenorrhea is Turner syndrome, while the most common cause of secondary amenorrhea is anovulation.

Amenorrhea may be dynamically evaluated by administering hormones that test the functional status of the endometrium. Administration of a progesterone derivative results in menses in women with adequate estrogenization (e.g., those with anovulation). If menses occur after administration of estrogen and progestin, this suggests a condition in which adequate estrogenization is not present (e.g., ovarian failure). If there is no bleeding with combined estrogen and progestin, this suggests either absence of the uterus or mechanical outflow obstruction.

Estrogen deficiency occurs in all women (menopause) and has many deleterious effects. Women with estrogen deficiency are at higher risk for osteoporosis. Estrogen was once felt to have beneficial cardiovascular effects. However, current studies show that the opposite is the case, and estrogen supplementation in menopausal women is only recommended for those with severe vasomotor symptoms and low cardiovascular risk, and then only for a short time (5 years or less) in most candidates.

Polycystic ovary syndrome is a common disorder of anovulation that is associated with hirsutism (increased facial hair), insulin resistance, and infertility. These patients are frequently obese, and are at higher future risk for developing type 2 diabetes. Insulin resistance and hyperandrogenism appear to be interrelated, with each affecting the other.

LIPIDS

Lipids are a group of naturally occurring molecules that include fats, waxes, sterols, fat-soluble vitamins, triglycerides, phospholipids, and other molecules. Lipids provide several essential functions to the body, despite lacking the glamour of, say, the hypothalamic–pituitary system. Yet, one exciting aspect of lipids is that they provide a storage depot of energy by placing a great deal of energy into a small package (9 kcal/g, as opposed to only 4 kcal/g for carbohydrate). Triglycerides (three fatty acids esterified to a glycerol molecule) are the main storage fuel and are denser and more anhydrous than glycogen, thereby occupying less space. Some birds are able to travel thousands of miles at a time because of extremely large and calorie-dense fat stores. For example, the average non-obese adult contains approximately 25–35 lb of fat; at a caloric density of 9 kcal/g, this results in approximately 100,000–150,000 kcal of total body stores. At an average expenditure of 2,000 kcal/day, this would last 50–75 days.

A Triglyceride Molecule

In addition, lipids are important structural parts of cell membranes (i.e., phospholipids). Cholesterol is not a fuel, but is necessary for synthesis of steroid hormones and in triglyceride metabolism. Bile acids, derived from cholesterol, act as detergents and help make nonpolar molecules soluble.

Lipids are also vital in signaling and may occur via activation of G protein-coupled or nuclear receptors, and molecules from several different lipid categories have been identified as signaling molecules and cellular messengers.

Although not a "classical" endocrine system, lipid metabolism is closely integrated with endocrine disorders (due to the effect of other endocrine disorders on lipid metabolism) and is thus often relegated to the endocrinologist for management. As we will see, many lipid disorders are associated with type 2 diabetes and metabolic syndrome.

LIPOPROTEINS

Lipids are organic molecules that are typically hydrophobic (meaning that they do not mix well with water). By themselves, they do not travel well in the bloodstream, so they require some type of "carrier protein" (just as many hormones do). Lipoproteins are carrier proteins that transport these hydrophobic lipid molecules in the plasma. They consist of a nonpolar lipid (triglycerides and cholesterol esters) core with an outer shell of more polar molecules (cholesterol, phospholipids, and apolipoproteins).

The four major lipoproteins in humans include chylomicrons, very low-density lipoproteins (VLDL), low-density lipoproteins (LDL), and high-density lipoproteins (HDL).

Chylomicrons are very large compared to the other proteins but are also the least dense (kind of like the "gas giant" planets Jupiter or Saturn in our solar system), consisting mainly of triglycerides (90%), and are therefore very energy rich. They transport dietary triglyceride from the gut into the lymphatics. They float to the top of plasma, forming a whitish "cream" layer. Triglycerides are removed from the chylomicrons by the

enzyme lipoprotein lipase, which yields triglyceride plus chylomicron remnants. Deficiency in lipoprotein lipase results in severe hypertriglyceridemia.

VLDL are next in size and consist chiefly of triglycerides, although they have less triglyceride than chylomicrons. They are important in the endogenous triglyceride pathway, transporting triglycerides made in the liver. As with chylomicrons, lipoprotein lipase removes triglyceride from VLDL, resulting in triglyceride plus intermediate-density lipoproteins (IDL).

LDL (also called β-lipoproteins) are cholesterol rich and are a result of the degradation of VLDL. As opposed to chylomicrons and VLDL, which transport triglycerides to lymphatics for energy, LDL transport cholesterol to peripheral tissues. They are much smaller than VLDL and chylomicrons and are taken up by LDL receptors. Increased LDL cholesterol is associated with premature atherosclerosis and is what is referred to by lay persons as "bad" cholesterol.

HDL (also called α-lipoproteins) are the smallest in size and contain only 20% cholesterol, the rest being phospholipid and apolipoproteins. They are the densest lipoproteins and are important in removing excess cholesterol from peripheral tissues. Increased levels of this "good" cholesterol are associated with a decreased incidence of atherosclerosis; decreased levels correlate with increased atherosclerosis. Some people have an inherited deficiency of HDL, making them much more prone to atherosclerotic events.

Apolipoproteins are small protein components that are part of the lipoprotein structure. Some act as ligands (binding sites) for receptors; others act as enzyme cofactors. Others provide structural integrity to the lipoprotein. Five classes exist in humans: A, B, C, D, and E.

The apo-A class of apolipoproteins is a major component of HDL and, to a lesser degree, chylomicrons and VLDL. The apo-B class is found in all lipoproteins except HDL. The major protein is apo-B-100, which is the ligand for binding LDL to its receptor. Excess of B-100-containing lipoproteins such as LDL is undesirable because these molecules are atherogenic. HDL, which does not contain apo-B, is antiatherogenic.

The apo-C apolipoproteins are primary components of VLDL and chylomicrons. Apo-D is found only in HDL and helps transfer cholesterol from HDL to apo-B-rich lipoproteins (e.g., LDL) in exchange for triglyceride. The cholesterol is then taken to the liver where it is disposed. The apo-E lipoproteins are receptor ligands for VLDL, chylomicron remnants, and IDL.

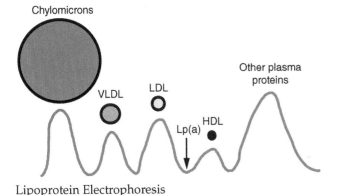

Lipoprotein Electrophoresis

Lipoprotein(a) or Lp(a) is a unique lipoprotein comprised of LDL attached to a protein, apoprotein(a). Lp(a) appears to inhibit thrombus (clot) dissolution and is atherogenic. High levels are clearly linked to premature atherosclerotic disease. Those with increased Lp(a) often respond poorly to drug therapy; nicotinic acid (niacin) seems to be the best treatment available.

HOW THE BODY OBTAINS LIPIDS

Triglycerides and cholesterol may be obtained either from diet (the exogenous lipid pathway) or from the degradation of lipid-rich lipoproteins (the endogenous lipid pathway). In addition, the body can synthesize cholesterol from smaller molecules. About half of the bile acids excreted into the small intestine are also "recycled" to be used as cholesterol again.

In the exogenous lipid pathway, dietary cholesterol is absorbed by the intestine and is incorporated into chylomicrons (which are made chiefly of triglyceride). Chylomicrons then go into the lymphatic system and then the bloodstream, where the enzyme lipoprotein lipase breaks the chylomicron into triglyceride and a chylomicron remnant, which contains cholesterol ester. The liver then assimilates the chylomicron remnant where free cholesterol is isolated.

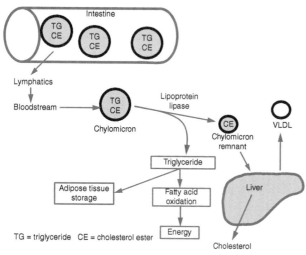

Exogenous Lipid Pathway

In the endogenous pathway, triglyceride- and cholesterol-rich VLDL is secreted by the liver, which is converted to triglyceride and IDL, again by lipoprotein lipase. HDL is also involved in this process. IDL is then converted to LDL, which is taken up by tissues with an LDL receptor.

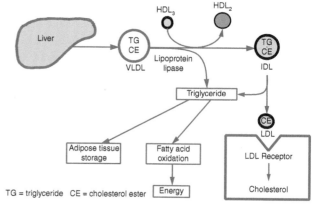

Endogenous Lipid Pathway

Cholesterol may also be made from acetate via a complex series of reactions. The most important step is the conversion of HMG-CoA to mevalonate by the enzyme HMG-CoA reductase. Increased cholesterol levels result in feedback inhibition of HMG-CoA reductase, thus decreasing synthesis.

HDL cholesterol is important in the reverse cholesterol pathway. Small, primordial HDL particles (nascent HDL) are secreted by the liver and intestines. Apolipoproteins bind to this immature HDL, and free cholesterol is acquired from cells, forming a slightly more advanced, small, cholesterol-poor, spherical HDL (HDL$_3$). Cholesterol is then attached to this HDL molecule by the enzyme lecithin-cholesterol acyltransferase (LCAT). The cholesterol molecules become more nonpolar, resulting in migration to the core and enlargement of the particle. This, along with transfer of apolipoprotein, cholesterol,

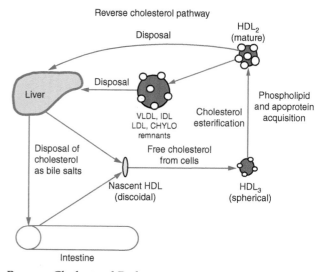

Reverse Cholesterol Pathway

and phospholipid from the delipidation of VLDL, results in a "mature" HDL particle (HDL_2). The excess cholesterol is then transferred to the apo-B-rich lipoproteins (LDL, VLDL, IDL, and chylomicron remnants), where they dispose of cholesterol in the liver, with excretion of the excess cholesterol as bile salts. Patients with low HDL levels therefore have decreased cholesterol removal and have an increased risk of atherosclerosis.

PRIMARY VERSUS SECONDARY DYSLIPIDEMIAS

Primary disorders are inherited, either as a specific gene mutation (e.g., primary hypercholesterolemia) or as a polygenic disorder (e.g., familial combined hyperlipidemia (FCHL)).

Primary hyperlipidemias traditionally were classified according to something called the Fredrickson classification, which characterizes lipid disorders according to the appearance (phenotype) of serum in a test tube after centrifugation. While seemingly quaint, this simple method remains very useful in the classification of primary lipid disorders, and it is useful to learn at least the most common lipid phenotypes. While you probably will not be looking at serum in test tubes (unless you become a clinical chemist), the concepts are useful in understanding pathophysiology. Remember that Fredrickson phenotypes may refer to either primary or secondary dyslipidemias and do not make references to the cause.

Although it seems intimidating, all it really takes to master the Fredrickson classification is to learn how lipoproteins look in serum. Chylomicrons are the least dense lipoproteins and always float to the top of plasma (think of our "gas giant" analogy; Saturn would float on water if a body of water sufficiently large to contain it existed). Since they contain lots of hydrophobic molecules (mostly triglyceride), they have a very milky, turbid appearance. VLDL is denser than chylomicrons, but mixed with the bottom layer and does not float to the top. Since VLDL contains a large number of triglycerides, they also create a somewhat turbid appearance. HDL and LDL are clear and are virtually indistinguishable to the naked eye from normal plasma.

Secondary dyslipidemias are caused by diseases interfering with lipoprotein metabolism, and may also be classified according to the Fredrickson subtypes; some secondary hyperlipidemias are more common than their primary counterparts. A common secondary disorder

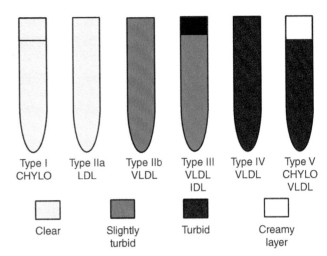

Fredrickson Phenotypes in Hyperlipidemia

is type IV or V hyperlipidemia associated with insulin resistance and type 2 diabetes. Hypothyroidism is also a very common contributor and may result in significant LDL elevation (type IIa).

The most common primary dyslipidemia is FCHL (Fredrickson type IIb) and occurs in about 1 in 100 persons. It is typically manifested as moderate elevations of both triglyceride (VLDL) and LDL cholesterol. The incidence of atherogenesis is increased; FCHL accounts for one-third to one-half of familial causes of CHD and 10% of cases of premature CHD. The type IIb phenotype also may occur as a secondary dyslipidemia (frequently with diabetes).

Familial hypercholesterolemia (Fredrickson phenotype IIa) is another common dyslipidemia. The heterozygous (one gene present) state is most common (1 in 500), resulting in elevated LDL and typical onset of coronary artery disease between ages 40 and 50. The homozygous (both genes present) state occurs in 1 per 1,000,000 patients; LDL levels are grossly elevated and coronary disease often begins between ages 10 and 20. The primary variety of type IIa is caused by an inherited defect in the LDL receptor, resulting in increased LDL and atherosclerosis. As with most dyslipidemias, secondary causes may occur; the most common secondary cause of type IIa is hypothyroidism.

Drug therapy may be effective for those with heterozygous type IIa disease. Homozygotes, however, respond poorly to conventional drug therapy, since there are very few functional LDL receptors; liver transplantation provides these functional receptors and offers the best hope of prolonging life in these individuals. Some patients may be treated with lipid apheresis, in which LDL is removed from serum; this procedure takes several hours and must be performed every 2 or 3 weeks, and availability is limited to certain lipid clinics at large medical centers. A new drug, lomitapide (a microsomal triglyceride transfer protein inhibitor), has been approved for use in the United States in adults with homozygous FH. Mipomersin is another new drug that inhibits gene expression of apo-B and requires a weekly subcutaneous injection.

Familial hypertriglyceridemia (type IV hyperlipidemia) is also a common disorder affecting approximately 1% of persons. This is a disorder of increased VLDL resulting in moderate to severe hypertriglyceridemia. The most common secondary cause of type IV is type 2 diabetes mellitus. Insulin plays a role in triglyceride removal, and impaired insulin action results in decreased clearance and hypertriglyceridemia.

Chylomicronemia syndrome or type V hyperlipidemia results from the increased accumulation of both VLDL and chylomicrons, resulting in severe hypertriglyceridemia. It is unusual as a primary lipid disorder and usually associated with a secondary cause (such as type 2 diabetes or glucocorticoid use).

Lipoprotein phenotypes are not always static; they may shift from one to another. For example, persons with poorly controlled diabetes often shift from type IV to V and back again after the diabetes is controlled.

PHYSICAL FINDINGS IN HYPERLIPIDEMIA

Many physical findings are present in patients with hyperlipidemia. Cholesterol accumulations called tendon xanthomas (areas of tendon thickening) may be seen in the extensor tendons (e.g., hand, patellar and Achilles areas) in those with severe hypercholesterolemia. They sometimes go away after cholesterol levels have been normalized. Eruptive xanthomas are seen in severe hypertriglyceridemia. These occur on the buttocks and over extensor surfaces of the arms and legs. They are pustular lesions that wax and wane with hypertriglyceridemia.

Corneal arcus is a whitish band on the outer cornea of the eye near the limbus. It is normal in elderly individuals but may indicate hypercholesterolemia in younger patients.

Xanthelasma is the yellowish plaques seen near the eyelids. They are commonly seen in hypercholesterolemia but are nonspecific, as many with this finding have no lipid disorder.

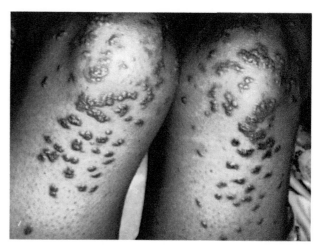

Eruptive Xanthomas

Lipemia retinalis is seen in those with severe hypertriglyceridemia (usually 3,000 mg/dL or greater). It is a whitish discoloration of the retinal vessels due to lipemic blood.

CONSEQUENCES OF HYPERLIPIDEMIA

Like diabetes mellitus, coronary artery disease is a major source of morbidity and mortality and a major expense to the health care system. As mentioned, LDL cholesterol elevation in particular leads to increased risk of atherosclerosis. Elevations in HDL cholesterol are actually protective against atherosclerosis. VLDL cholesterol elevation is usually associated with hypertriglyceridemia.

Severe hypertriglyceridemia may cause acute pancreatitis, with nausea, vomiting, and abdominal pain. Repeated attacks may result in chronic pancreatitis, pancreatic insufficiency, and even death. The significance of mild hypertriglyceridemia is less obvious. In the past, it was felt that isolated hypertriglyceridemia was not a risk factor for cardiovascular disease, and modest hypertriglyceridemia (<500 mg/dL) was tolerated and even ignored. However, hypertriglyceridemia does lower HDL levels, thus potentiating cardiac risk in this manner. It is also now recognized that persons with hypertriglyceridemia develop a denser, more atherogenic form of LDL; normalization of triglycerides decreases its concentration. It is now recommended that triglyceride levels be normalized if possible through diet or medication.

THERAPY OF HYPERLIPIDEMIA

Drug therapy should never be initiated based on an elevated isolated total cholesterol level; a lipoprotein profile should be obtained to identify specific abnormalities. Total cholesterol may be elevated because of elevated LDL, VLDL, or even HDL. For example, LDL elevation may be treated with one type of drug, while those with VLDL cholesterol elevation might require another type of drug (and some drugs, such as bile acid sequestrants, actually can worsen VLDL cholesterol (triglycerides), making the condition worse). Those with high total cholesterol (with normal LDL and triglycerides) due to high HDL require no treatment; indeed, this abnormality appears to confer protection against atherosclerotic disease.

Diet is a cornerstone of therapy that (like in diabetes) unfortunately, may be quite difficult for the patient. Many persons who are willing to take a lipid-lowering medication are unwilling to make sufficient dietary modifications. Consultation with a registered dietitian is recommended to help meal planning; this service can be obtained at an outpatient center or lipid clinic. This is especially important since many patients with hyperlipidemia also have diabetes.

If dietary therapy fails, lipid-lowering medication should be used. The most commonly used drugs are the HMG-CoA reductase inhibitors (often called "statins"). These drugs are derived from fungal fermentation products and are competitive inhibitors of HMG-CoA reductase, the rate-limiting step in cholesterol biosynthesis. They are extremely effective at reducing LDL cholesterol, are easily taken orally and are well tolerated in most cases. They are much less useful for the treatment of hypertriglyceridemia. Examples include lovastatin, atorvastatin, and simvastatin. These drugs rarely cause myositis and hepatic transaminase elevation, which may require discontinuation or dose reduction.

Fibric acid derivatives (fibrates) are primarily used in the treatment of hypertriglyceridemia. They are less effective than statins for isolated LDL elevation. Fibrates work by increasing VLDL and chylomicron clearance and inhibiting VLDL production. Currently available drugs include gemfibrozil and fenofibrate.

Resins or bile acid sequestrants are charged molecules that bind bile acids in the intestine. Since much of the body's cholesterol is derived from the recirculating "pool" of bile acids, diminishing the size of the pool decreases the body's cholesterol; this bile acid–resin complex is then eliminated in the stool. Common side effects of resins include constipation and bloating. Resins should be taken alone, since they are highly charged molecules which may bind and impair the absorption of other medications. For poorly understood reasons, resins may increase VLDL synthesis and therefore exacerbate pre-existing hypertriglyceridemia, and should be avoided in patients with triglyceride problems. Available resins include cholestyramine, colesevelam, and colestipol. These lipid-lowering medications are not systemically absorbed by the body. Interestingly, resins have a very modest effect on lowering glucose levels in diabetes mellitus (0.5% average reduction in hemoglobin A_{1c}), although they are not commonly used for this purpose. The mechanism of action of their glucose-lowering properties is not fully understood.

Cholesterol absorption inhibitors specifically act at the level of the brush border of the small intestine by preventing the absorption of cholesterol. The currently available drug is ezetimibe. An advantage is that, like bile acid sequestrants, it is not systemically absorbed by the body (and thus generally free of systemic side effects as may be seen with other drugs). In addition, it appears to act synergistically with statin drugs. While well tolerated, it has a more modest effect on LDL reduction than reductase inhibitors, and there is much less evidence for reduction in cardiovascular events than for other drugs.

Nicotinic acid (niacin, vitamin B-3) is required for normal metabolism but has potent lipid-lowering characteristics in large doses. (It is not related to nicotine, a psychoactive alkaloid found in tobacco and pesticides.) Niacin has been used for many years and is an excellent treatment for both LDL cholesterol elevation and hypertriglyceridemia. Modest HDL cholesterol elevation also occurs with niacin therapy.

Niacin, however, is the "Dr Jekyll and Mr Hyde" of lipid-lowering medications. The Dr Jekyll form is beneficial and helps lower LDL and triglyceride levels; indeed, niacin can be a very effective medication. But the Mr Hyde side of niacin is seen in its many side effects. The most frequent is cutaneous flushing, similar to the menopausal "hot flash." This reaction is caused by prostaglandins and often averted by giving inhibitors of prostaglandin synthesis (e.g., aspirin) shortly before dosing.

Niacin may worsen insulin resistance and raise blood glucose, and must be used with caution in individuals with impaired glucose tolerance or diabetes mellitus.

Ironically, such individuals are often the ones with severe hypertriglyceridemia who need treatment most—a tough situation. One advantage of niacin is its low cost for generic forms. However, this is less important now that many reductase inhibitors (statins) and fibrates are on the generic market; it is sort of a "niche" drug for special situations (which are relatively uncommon). But, in the right patient population, it can be very effective.

Many years ago, it was observed that atherosclerotic disease is low among Greenland Eskimos consuming large amounts of seafood; it was discovered that fish oils contain long-chain polyunsaturated omega-3 fatty acids: eicosapentaenoic acid (EPA) and docosahexaenoic acid (DHA). Omega-3 fatty acids significantly lower VLDL cholesterol (and therefore triglyceride) levels in hyperlipidemic patients. Fish oil therapy causes little or no change in those with normal lipids or with isolated cholesterol elevation. They also appear to have anti-atherogenic effects that are independent of the lipid-lowering effects, possibly due to their effect on prostaglandin metabolism. They may be of use in patients with severe hypertriglyceridemia unresponsive to fibrates and/or niacin. They increase hepatic glucose production and must be used with caution in those with diabetes. Omega-3 fatty acids can be obtained as an over-the-counter supplement or as a pharmacologic preparation (esterified fish oils).

Pharmacologic Agents Used in Hyperlipidemia

Drug Type	Major Use	Possible Side Effects
HMG-CoA reductase inhibitors (statins)	LDL reduction	Transaminase elevation, myositis (rare)
Fibric acid derivatives	TG reduction	Transaminase elevation, myositis (rare)
Nicotinic acid (niacin)	LDL and TG reduction	Flushing, worsening of glucose tolerance, diarrhea
Bile acid sequestrants	LDL reduction	Constipation, TG elevation, potential interference with drug absorption
Cholesterol absorption inhibitor (ezetimibe)	LDL reduction	Rare; bloating, diarrhea, headache occasionally seen
Omega-3 fatty acids	TG reduction	Worsening of glucose tolerance

REVIEW QUESTIONS

1. A 47-year old male presents for general health screening. He has not been to a physician in several years. He has a history of smoking in the past but quit 5 years ago; his father died at age 58 of a myocardial infarction. He is noted to have a total serum cholesterol of 257 mg/dL on a routine chemistry profile. He is overweight with a BMI of 32 m/kg² and normotensive (blood pressure 129/80 mm). Physical examination is unremarkable.
Regarding the management of his cholesterol level:
a. He should start pravastatin, 10 mg once daily
b. He should see a registered dietitian regarding weight loss
c. He should have an exercise stress test
d. He needs to have a lipid profile to determine which lipoprotein fractions are abnormal
e. He should start cholestyramine or colesevelam

(d) He needs to have a lipid profile before any intervention is taken regarding his lipids. Although his total cholesterol is elevated, this could be from deleterious elevations (LDL or VLDL (triglycerides)) or beneficial ones (HDL). Medications are inappropriate without this information; bile acid sequestrants might even worsen hypercholesterolemia due to triglyceride (VLDL) elevation. While there is nothing wrong with referring an overweight man to the dietitian (b), it should not be done specifically to address the lipids without further information. Similarly, a cardiac stress test (c) might be appropriate in a former smoker with family history of cardiac disease, but it should be for those reasons and not lipids without further information.

2. A 49-year old woman with a history of poorly controlled diabetes mellitus presents for an annual visit.

She is hypertensive with a BMI of 34 kg/m^2 and demonstrates poor control with a HbA$_{1c}$ of 8.9%. Her LDL cholesterol is 97 mg/dL on pravastatin, 20 mg daily, but triglycerides are elevated at 477 mg/dL. Her medications include metformin and linagliptin.

Regarding her triglycerides, she would benefit most now from which one of the following?

a. Addition of nicotinic acid

b. Beginning an exercise program and consulting with a registered dietitian

c. Replacing pravastatin with fenofibrate

d. Beginning insulin

e. Adding a sulfonylurea

(d) This patient likely has type IV hyperlipidemia due to poor glycemic control; insulin activity is necessary for proper functioning of lipoprotein lipase, necessary for clearing of both VLDL and chylomicrons. With a hemoglobin A$_{1c}$ of almost 9%, only insulin therapy will bring her glucose levels down sufficiently to help this problem. While diet and exercise (b) should also be undertaken, it will take some time for this to have significant effect. If her BMI does substantially decrease, then she might be able to come off insulin. Addition of sulfonylureas (e) or any other non-insulin agent will not achieve the desired outcome. Niacin (a) at therapeutic doses may decrease TG levels, but will invariably worsen her glucose control now. Fenofibrate (c) is a better option than niacin, but still should only be considered once her diabetes control has improved.

Disorders of Multiple Endocrine Glands and Paraneoplastic Syndromes

REVIEW

Let us review what we learned in the last lecture. Lipids provide several essential functions to the body. Their most important function is to provide long-term energy storage. Lipids are also important as precursors for hormones and structural components of cell membranes.

There are four major lipoproteins in humans. These include chylomicrons, very low-density lipoproteins (VLDL), low-density lipoproteins (LDL), and high-density lipoproteins (HDL). Chylomicrons are the least dense and float to the top of plasma if left standing in a test tube; they consist chiefly of triglycerides. VLDL lipoproteins are also very rich in triglycerides and carry cholesterol as well. LDL is very cholesterol rich and is an important factor in atherogenesis. HDL is the smallest lipoprotein and is important in removing cholesterol from peripheral tissues. Increased HDL is thus inversely correlated with atherosclerosis. Apolipoproteins are the building blocks of lipoproteins.

There are several important pathways of lipid metabolism in humans. The endogenous lipid pathway is how the body obtains lipids from the diet. In this system, triglyceride-rich chylomicrons are absorbed by the lymphatic system. Cholesterol is later isolated from chylomicron remnants by the liver. In the endogenous pathway, the liver secretes triglyceride and cholesterol-rich VLDL particles, which are then converted to free triglyceride and other particles by lipoprotein lipase. LDL is formed, which is taken up by tissues with an LDL receptor.

In addition, the body makes its own cholesterol. The rate-limiting step of cholesterol biosynthesis is catalyzed by the enzyme HMG-CoA reductase.

Lipoprotein disorders may be classified as primary or secondary. Primary lipid disorders are inherited. Secondary disorders are caused by another disorder, such as diabetes. Both types of lipid disorders are sometimes classified according to the Fredrickson scheme, which groups lipid phenotypes according to the appearance of serum in a test tube.

The most common primary dyslipidemia is familial combined (type IIb) hyperlipidemia. The second most common is familial hypercholesterolemia (type IIa). Those with heterozygous type IIa disease often develop premature atherosclerosis by the ages of 40–50; those with homozygous disease may develop disease in the second or third decades of life. Other types of primary hyperlipidemia are uncommon.

Diabetes is a common cause of secondary hyperlipidemia, frequently resulting in type IV and type V hyperlipidemia due to acquired defects in triglyceride metabolism. Hypothyroidism frequently results in type IIa hyperlipidemia.

Multiple clinical studies have demonstrated decreased morbidity and mortality from coronary artery disease in aggressive therapy of patients with hyperlipidemia. Atherosclerosis is most commonly linked to elevated LDL cholesterol, although hypertriglyceridemia has also been shown to play a role in atherosclerosis. Many patients with hypertriglyceridemia also have diabetes.

The first line of treatment in hyperlipidemia is diet therapy, which may be difficult for some patients. Multiple pharmacologic agents are also available. The most useful are the HMG-CoA reductase inhibitors (statins), which inhibit cholesterol synthesis and result in dramatic lowering of LDL cholesterol; they are less useful in lowering triglycerides. Cholesterol absorption inhibitors (ezetimibe) have a modest effect on LDL lowering, and appear to be synergistic with statins. Fibric acid derivatives (fibrates) are useful in the treatment of hypertriglyceridemia. The vitamin nicotinic acid (niacin) is a useful drug in the treatment of both hypercholesterolemia and hypertriglyceridemia, but use is limited by its frequent unpleasant side effects; extended-release preparations can lessen these to some extent. Resins or bile acid sequestrants are useful in patients with mild to moderate LDL cholesterol elevations but may actually worsen hypertriglyceridemia.

POLYENDOCRINE SYNDROMES

We have thus far discussed endocrine disorders specific to the organ system. This lecture attempts to "put it all together" and discuss disorders that affect more than one endocrine system—the polyendocrine disorders. Lastly, I will discuss the so-called ectopic endocrine or paraneoplastic syndromes—endocrine disorders resulting from secretion of hormones from non-endocrine system tumors.

These disorders involve more than one endocrine system and may be divided into (1) the immunoendocrine syndromes and (2) the multiple endocrine neoplasia (MEN) syndromes. With few exceptions, the former are disorders of endocrine deficiency while the latter are syndromes of endocrine excess. They are commonly confused with one another, although they are fundamentally different disorders. Also, while the immunoendocrine syndromes are very common, MEN syndromes are rare.

The immunoendocrine disorders are autoimmune syndromes that affect multiple endocrine organs. The first was described in 1926 by Schmidt, who reported autopsy findings in two patients with "a two-gland illness" (adrenal insufficiency and hypothyroidism). This syndrome may also be associated with other disorders and is sometimes called Schmidt's syndrome or polyglandular autoimmune syndrome type II (PGA II). It is important to be aware of these syndromes, since a patient with one autoimmune endocrine disorder may be at risk for developing further endocrine disorders. They are genetically transmitted; therefore, genetic counseling and surveillance of family members is important.

Type II polyglandular syndrome (PGA II) is the most common of the endocrine deficiency syndromes. It involves the occurrence of two or more of the following autoimmune endocrine disorders in the same individual: Addison's disease, Hashimoto's thyroiditis, Graves' disease, type 1 diabetes mellitus, and/or primary gonadal failure. (Note that Graves' disease is unique because it is an autoimmune disorder of hormonal excess; the others are deficiency syndromes.) Pernicious anemia and vitiligo also may be seen.

In order to qualify, the disorders must be autoimmune; that is, adrenal failure due to histoplasmosis, hypothyroidism due to thyroidectomy, and type 2 diabetes do not count.

The individual diseases are identical to—and are treated just like—those which occur individually. One disease may commonly exacerbate another, however (e.g., adrenal insufficiency aggravates hypoglycemic responsiveness in type 1 diabetics and hyperthyroidism aggravates adrenal insufficiency and diabetes control), so it is important to recognize if multiple disorders are present.

The type I syndrome is much less common and primarily seen in children. It is usually associated with Addison's disease, mucocutaneous candidiasis, and hypoparathyroidism. Other endocrine abnormalities are rarely seen (much less commonly than in PGA II) and include hypothyroidism, Graves' disease, gonadal failure, and diabetes mellitus.

Multiple endocrine neoplasia (MEN)

MEN syndromes are associated with multiple endocrine tumors, benign and malignant, which result in syndromes of hormone excess. Hormone deficiency may occasionally occur as the result of destructive effects of a large tumor (e.g., pituitary). MEN syndromes are uncommon and are divided into two broad categories: MEN I and MEN IIa/IIb.

MEN I is characterized by the "three Ps"—pituitary, pancreatic islet, and parathyroid tumors. Two or more tumors in the same individual are diagnostic for MEN. Hyperparathyroidism is the most common manifestation, occurring in over 95% of those affected. By age 40, almost all carrying the gene have hypercalcemia.

Pancreatic islet cell tumors are the second most common manifestation, occurring in up to 80% of patients. The tumors are typically multicentric, and therefore surgical cure is difficult. Pharmacologic treatment of the hormone excess is often required.

The most common MEN I pancreatic tumor is gastrinoma, leading to Zollinger–Ellison syndrome (gastric acid hypersecretion), multiple peptic ulcers, and diarrhea. Serum gastrin levels are usually elevated. Treatment includes histamine-2 (H_2) antagonists (e.g., cimetidine, ranitidine) and/or proton pump inhibitors (omeprazole, esomeprazole, etc.), and gastrectomy may be required. Since the pancreatic peptide somatostatin (the same one made by the hypothalamus) inhibits gastrin secretion, the long-acting somatostatin analog octreotide may be useful.

Insulinoma is the second most common pancreatic tumor. This results in severe fasting hypoglycemia with inappropriately elevated serum insulin and C-peptide concentrations. Seizures and death may occur if untreated. As these tumors are usually multicentric, total pancreatectomy may be required.

Pituitary adenomas are the third most common manifestation and occur in over 50% of patients with MEN I. These include prolactin, growth hormone, and ACTH-secreting tumors, with the associated clinical manifestations. Tumors may also be nonfunctional and cause compressive symptoms if large enough.

Carcinoid tumors also may occur but are the least common tumor type. These produce large amounts of serotonin and cause severe flushing and diarrhea. Lipomas (subcutaneous and visceral) are also associated, but do not produce hormones.

MEN IIa is the association of medullary thyroid carcinoma with pheochromocytoma and, less commonly, hyperparathyroidism. Calcitonin levels are usually elevated in these patients. Pheochromocytoma presents with the typical manifestations of hypertension, tachycardia, headaches, hyperhidrosis, and cardiac arrhythmias. Clinical history and elevation of serum or urine catecholamines and metabolites typically establish the diagnosis. MRI or CT may localize the tumor. Hyperparathyroidism may also be present, although much less commonly than in MEN I (10–20% of MEN IIa as opposed to >90% of MEN I).

MEN type IIb is the combination of medullary thyroid carcinoma, pheochromocytoma, multiple mucosal neuromas, and a characteristic marfanoid habitus (long, thin body habitus with arachnodactyly). Hyperparathyroidism is not seen in this disorder.

PARANEOPLASTIC SYNDROMES

These are also called ectopic or "out of place" endocrine syndromes, since the hormones are produced by tumors of non-endocrine origin. For example, insulin produced by a pancreatic insulinoma is not a paraneoplastic syndrome since the tumor normally makes this substance. These disorders were first recognized by the association of hypercalcemia with certain malignancies. In this lecture we will discuss the most common paraneoplastic syndromes.

The most common ectopic syndrome is hypercalcemia and is usually caused by secretion of a substance called PTH-related peptide (PTH-rP). While PTH-rP does have human physiological significance (e.g., in normal breast and placental development), it does not normally rise to sufficient concentrations in normal health to cause hypercalcemia. This syndrome is termed humoral hypercalcemia of malignancy (HHM). Another type of paraneoplastic hypercalcemia is called local osteolytic hypercalcemia (LOH), and accounts for most of the remaining patients with paraneoplastic hypercalcemia. LOH is caused by osteoclast-activating factors (OAFs) that cause bone destruction (lysis) and hypercalcemia. Very rarely, some hematologic malignancies (lymphomas) may produce calcitriol, resulting in a type of vitamin D-dependent hypercalcemia.

How do we distinguish HHM from primary hyperparathyroidism? By measuring PTH and PTH-rP. In HHM, native PTH levels will be suppressed, because of normal feedback on the parathyroids, while the level of PTH-rP is elevated. In primary hyperparathyroidism, PTH levels are high, while PTH-rP levels are low. HHM is very aggressive, while primary hyperparathyroidism typically presents with mild hypercalcemia that progresses slowly over several years.

Syndrome of inappropriate antidiuretic hormone (SIADH) is the next most common paraneoplastic syndrome. It is usually obvious that this is a paraneoplastic syndrome, since tumors of the native gland do not produce this condition.

Cushing's syndrome due to ectopic ACTH secretion is the third most common ectopic syndrome. Since the tumor (usually small cell lung carcinoma) is typically quite aggressive, the clinical appearance may evolve over weeks, as compared to the relatively indolent Cushing's disease due to pituitary tumors, which may take months to years to notice. Iatrogenic Cushing's or Cushing's syndrome due to adrenal tumors can be easily differentiated from ectopic ACTH syndrome, since ACTH levels are low in the former two. If the distinction between Cushing's disease and ectopic ACTH syndrome is not obvious, petrosal sinus (blood vessels draining the pituitary) sampling can be done. With Cushing's disease, petrosal sinus ACTH is greater than peripheral blood ACTH. The high-dose dexamethasone suppression test can also be useful, if desired. A less common type of ectopic ACTH syndrome associated with bronchial carcinoids is less aggressive, and may be harder to distinguish from Cushing's disease.

Treatment of paraneoplastic syndromes is directed at the primary tumor, if possible. If tumor shrinkage occurs, hormone secretion also diminishes and the syndrome improves. Specific antagonist therapy may be required in conjunction with antitumor therapy, as some tumors do not respond well to therapy.

Hypercalcemia of malignancy due to PTH-rP is best treated with inhibitors of bone resorption (bisphosphonates such as zoledronic acid and pamidronate are effective). Salmon calcitonin is a weak antagonist and is useful only in mild cases. More potent but toxic antiresorptive agents include gallium nitrate.

Patients with hypercalcemia of malignancy are usually quite dehydrated and normal saline administration promotes calciuresis. Radiation therapy may benefit those with LOH. Those with hypercalcemia due to immunologic factors or calcitriol respond to glucocorticoids.

SIADH is usually treated with fluid restriction and management of the underlying disease. In refractory cases, demeclocycline, which produces ADH resistance (and thus a state of nephrogenic diabetes insipidus), may be used. Intravenous vasopressin antagonists (conivaptan and tolvaptan) are also used in selected hospitalized patients with severe hyponatremia.

Ectopic ACTH syndrome may be treated with drugs that inhibit adrenal steroid synthesis, such as mitotane, ketoconazole, and aminoglutethimide. The aldosterone antagonists spironolactone and eplerenone aid in correcting the metabolic effects of mineralocorticoid excess, such as hypokalemia. If these measures are unsuccessful, bilateral adrenalectomy may be required. These patients typically have a poor prognosis.

REVIEW QUESTIONS

1. Which endocrine excess disorder would not be seen in any of the MEN syndromes?
   a. Acromegaly
   b. Cushing's disease
   c. Graves' disease
   d. Insulinoma
   e. Pheochromocytoma

   (c) Graves' disease is an autoimmune disorder and not a neoplastic disorder. Acromegaly, Cushing's disease and insulinoma can be seen with MEN I; pheochromocytoma is associated with MEN IIa and/or IIb.

2. The most common manifestation of MEN I is:
   a. Acromegaly
   b. Primary hyperparathyroidism
   c. Pheochromocytoma
   d. Hypothyroidism
   e. Insulinoma

   (b) This is by far the most common manifestation of MEN I, being present in 95% of patients. Pheochromocytoma (c) is seen in MEN IIa/b, not I. Hypothyroidism is not a component of MEN syndromes.

3. Which of the following is not a paraneoplastic syndrome?
   a. Cushing's syndrome due to small cell lung carcinoma
   b. SIADH due to small cell lung carcinoma
   c. Hypercalcemia due to breast cancer
   d. Hypercalcitoninemia due to metastatic medullary thyroid cancer

   (d) The parafollicular (c) cells of the thyroid normally make calcitonin, so this is merely a manifestation of metastatic disease, and not a paraneoplastic syndrome.

Clinical Trials, Evidence-Based Medicine, and Reading the Literature

APPENDIX

Medicine used to be taught by learning from preceptors and doing what they did, by virtue of their experience. However, while experience is invaluable, in today's world we need to practice "evidence-based medicine." In other words, we need to back up our actions with robust, peer-reviewed literature. In this lecture I will deviate from endocrinology a bit and discuss some important statistical principles you should master so that you know how to read the medical literature and understand the basic "lingo" of evidence-based medicine.

One example I will discuss later (in the section on glucose metabolism) is that, for years, we did not know if treating diabetes mellitus aggressively decreased the rate of complications. The Diabetes Control and Complications Trial (DCCT), published in 1993, was a landmark study. Let us use this as an example of evidence-based medicine.

Among those volunteers who previously had exhibited no retinopathy, intensive control therapy reduced the adjusted mean risk of this complication by 76%. Among those who had mild retinopathy, intensive control therapy slowed the progression of retinopathy by 54% and reduced the development of severe nonproliferative retinopathy by 47%.

One fundamental lesson to take away from this trial is that one cannot simply extrapolate findings in one study to another population. For example, the DCCT only studied patients with type 1 diabetes. Can we assume that the reduction in complications can be applied to patients with type 2 diabetes as well (which is very important given the much greater number of patients with type 2)?

While it would be nice to do that, there might be differences in the two populations, which would prohibit this from being a valid comparison. To be robust, we need to do another study with the population of interest.

Also, notice that the reduction in complications only pertained to microvascular complications, and not

Other Major Findings in the DCCT

Albuminuria

Intensive control therapy reduced microalbuminuria (40 mg/day) by 39%.

Intensive control therapy reduced albuminuria (300 mg/day) by 54%.

Neuropathy

Intensive control therapy reduced clinical neuropathy by 60%.

Intensive control therapy reduced abnormal nerve conduction by 44%.

Intensive control therapy reduced abnormal autonomic nervous system function by 53%.

Nerve conduction velocities remained stable with intensive control therapy, but decreased with conventional therapy.

Severe hypoglycemia

The chief adverse event associated with intensive therapy was a 200–300% increase in severe hypoglycemia, which is statistically significant.

macrovascular (more about this later). While microvascular complications are important, we would also like to know if reduction in cardiovascular disease, stroke, hypertension, and so on (all macrovascular complications) would be seen. Since the study did not find those statistically significant, we cannot say for certain.

Another study, the United Kingdom Prospective Diabetes Study (UKPDS), was done. This study demonstrated similar findings to the DCCT regarding patients with type 2 diabetes, but did not find statistically significant results regarding macrovascular complications.

Major Landmark Lipid Trials

Study	Result
Framingham study (started 1948; ongoing, currently on third generation of participants)	Cholesterol levels are linked with long-term cardiovascular mortality in persons under age 50
Lipid Research Clinics—Coronary Primary Prevention Trial I (LRC-CPPT) (1984)	Patients treated with cholestyramine for several years had decrease in death from coronary disease and decrease in nonfatal myocardial infarction
Helsinki Heart Study (1980s)	Gemfibrozil reduced the incidence of coronary disease in men with hyperlipidemia
Familial Atherosclerosis Treatment Study (FATS)—1999	Reduction in LDL cholesterol in men resulted in decreased progression of coronary disease and incidence of cardiac events in high-risk men receiving lovastatin + colestipol or niacin + colestipol
St Thomas Atherosclerosis Regression Study (STARS) (1998)	Diet alone or diet + cholestyramine slowed progression and increased regression of coronary artery disease
Monitored Atherosclerosis Regression Study (MARS)—1990s	Lovastatin + diet decreased progression of coronary lesions in patients with coronary disease
Scandinavian Simvastatin Survival Study (1990s)	Simvastatin decreases the relative risk for death in patients with CAD
Cholesterol Lowering Atherosclerosis Study (1987)	Non-progression and regression of coronary lesions in those treated with colestipol + niacin

Another important group of trials discussed control of inpatients with diabetes. The first group of trials came out in 2000 and recommended inpatient control ranges of 80–110 mg/dL (4.4–6.1 mmol/L).

Eventually, this degree of control was determined to be too aggressive (as the cost of such rigorous control in the hospital was excessive hypoglycemia) and current recommendations are that glucose levels be kept at 140–180 mg/dL (7.7–9.9 mmol/L) in most cases.

Another important set of studies are the lipid trials, too many to discuss in this textbook. Summarized above are many of the major landmark trials throughout the years, although there are many others.

As discussed, the DCCT, which assessed the impact of intensive versus standard glycemic control in type 1 diabetes, did not find a significant difference in rates of cardiovascular events with intensive therapy during the main study period. However, long-term follow-up of those same patients in The Epidemiology of Diabetes Interventions and Complications Study (EDIC) found that those previously treated intensively had a significant 42% reduction in the risk of any cardiovascular event. The risk of nonfatal myocardial infarction, stroke, or death from cardiovascular disease was reduced by 57% in those previously assigned to intensive glycemic control.

SENSITIVITY, SPECIFICITY, AND PRETEST PROBABILITY

The availability of an increasing number of complex diagnostic tests, along with concerns over the rising costs of health care, has generated renewed interest in determining the most effective means of utilizing tests. Good clinical judgment requires that the physician choose tests in a cost-effective manner, so that the results lead to improved diagnosis and treatment.

When considering a test, the physician must determine whether the test is efficacious and sufficiently accurate, that no other test with acceptable efficacy is less hazardous or less expensive, and that this is the most appropriate time for ordering the test. As we shall see, practical use depends on many statistical factors.

One measure of the effectiveness of a test is the sensitivity and specificity. The sensitivity of any test is its ability to detect the disorder in patients who already have it. The specificity, on the other hand, is the ability of any test to exclude those patients who do not have it. Ideally we want our test to be high in both. But there is more to interpreting test results than just these two quantities.

Do not believe that if a test has a very high sensitivity and specificity, it will be useful in screening all patient populations and will always provide accurate information. Remember that sensitivity and specificity refer to the populations of patients either with (sensitivity) or without (specificity) disease; in real life, these populations will not be known. Instead, we are concerned about the significance of a positive or negative test result. (The positive predictive value (PPV) or negative predictive value (NPV), respectively.)

In 1763 mathematician Thomas Bayes demonstrated the manner in which the predictive value is influenced not only by the sensitivity/specificity but also by the "prior probability" (prevalence) of the disease. This is the principle of Bayes' Theorem, which demonstrates that the sensitivity and specificity of a diagnostic test are functions of the test itself and really do not depend on the prevalence of the disease, whereas the PPV and NPV do.

In any test, we may have any one of four outcomes:

Test Result	Disease Present	No Disease
Positive	True positive (TP) Power $(1 - \beta)$	False positive (FP) Type I error (α)
Negative	False negative (FN) Type II Error (β)	True negative (TN)

The SENSITIVITY of a test is an index of the capacity to detect an abnormality (i.e., be positive) in a population of patients having the disease. It is therefore the number of true positives over the total with the disease, or

$$SENSITIVITY = TP/(TP + FN)$$

The SPECIFICITY indicates the test's ability to exclude a normal subject (be negative) in that population *without* the disease and is defined as:

$$SPECIFICITY = TN/(TN + FP)$$

However, per Bayes' theorem, these are functions of the test itself, and these indices do not tell us what we really want to know: what does a positive (or negative) test result mean to you, the clinician (as you do not know which populations have disease and which do not)?

If we do some mathematical manipulation (as Bayes did in the 1700s), we arrive at the formula for PPV:

$$PPV = \frac{Sens}{Sens + Spec - 1 + \frac{1-Spec}{Prevalence}}$$

Notice that, while PPV depends on sensitivity and specificity, it also (as Bayes discovered) depends on the disease prevalence. Specifically, as prevalence increases, PPV increases; as prevalence decreases, so does PPV. (The opposite happens with NPV; as prevalence increases, NPV decreases, and vice versa.)

Let us do some sample calculations with a theoretical test with a sensitivity and specificity of 95%. This is a superb test and few real-world examples exist for this, but we will use it for our examples. Consider two populations of a million patients: one with disease prevalence of 5% and the other with 80%.

For the population with prevalence of 5%, it can be shown that the number of false positives (47,500, FP) equals those with the disease itself (47,500). So the PPV in this case is only 0.50, meaning that the probability of your patient having the disease if the test is positive is essentially a coin toss. So use your test results with caution in populations with low disease prevalence.

For the high prevalence population (80%), the converse is true; the false positives number only 10,000 with TP of 760,000, so the PPV rises to 0.99. So a positive result is most significant in populations with high prevalence rates.

What about the significance of a negative result (NPV)? It is the opposite. For the 5% group, FN = 2,500 and TN = 902,500, with an NPV of 0.997. So, you can be more confident that a negative result truly represents a negative disease state with a low prevalence. With the 80% group, there are 40,000 FN and 190,000 TN, with an NPV of 0.83. So the NPV went down with increasing disease prevalence.

It can be mathematically shown that PPV equals NPV at a disease prevalence of 50%; also, PPV falls off rapidly below a prevalence of 10%, while the same happens for NPV at prevalence over 90%. So interpret any test results with caution in populations with prevalence over 90% or under 10% (see graph):

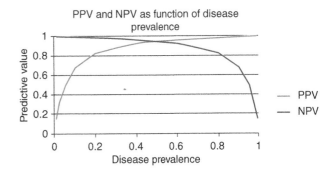

A common real world example: a positive treadmill stress test result in a 30-year-old healthy nonsmoking female likely represents a false positive (given that the pretest probability of cardiac disease in this population is extremely remote), while a negative result essentially excludes disease. In contrast, a positive result in a 90-year-old male with history of hypertension and diabetes likely confirms ischemia, while a negative result may represent a false negative and warrants further investigation. In other words, interpret your test results with the concept of "pretest probability" in mind and how it will affect your interpretation.

In summary, the ordering of diagnostic tests will become more cost-effective if you estimate the pretest probability, order the appropriate test, and properly integrate the test result with the available clinical information. A test will be helpful only if it provides information above and beyond what was previously available—that is, if it changes the probability of disease to cross the thresholds for decision-making. Tests should be ordered only if their incremental information will have a positive effect on patient care.

The price for missing a diagnosis should also be weighed along with the pretest probability, that is, you may go to great lengths to exclude angina pectoris; failure to quickly diagnose a more benign disease is not as worrisome. As private insurance and government play an increasing role in deciding medical care we need to be as effective as possible in the utilization of diagnostic testing.

Statistical significance: *p* value demystified

The "*p* value" is a fundamental concept of statistics and quoted in any work that uses statistical analyses to determine if a true difference between two groups exists. But what does it really mean?

p stands for probability—and, in statistical terms, refers to the probability that the measured difference between the two groups occurred purely by chance and not due to any true difference. Therefore, the *lower* the *p* value, the better.

Let us examine the simple exercise of tossing two different quarter-dollar coins 10 times. In any statistical analysis we must have a *null hypothesis* (H_0), which states that there is *no* difference between the populations that the two groups represent (in this case, all the quarters in the world). The *alternative hypothesis* (H_1) is a rejection of the null, and states that there *is* a difference between the two populations represented by the quarters. Usually, in biomedical studies, we are looking for a difference between the two groups—for example, one drug is more

effective than another, a certain intervention detected colon cancer earlier—so we often *want* to reject H_0.

In our quarter-flipping example, the null hypothesis maintains that there is *no* difference between the two quarters (and we should obtain similar results with each); H_1 states that there is a difference (i.e., the quarters differ to the extent that heads or tails will come up more often than expected). Remember that these hypotheses refer to the *populations* of all entities they represent and not just the *samples*.

We try the first quarter and flip it 10 times: 6 heads, 4 tails (*p* of heads = 0.6). The probability of tossing heads on any single throw is 0.5; therefore, we expect heads approximately one-half of the time. With 10 flips, 0.6 seems fairly close to 0.5.

But, for a second quarter, we obtain 10 heads. We scratch our heads and think of what the probability of tossing 10 straight heads would be; it is $(0.5)^{10}$ or approximately 0.001. This means that, if the quarter is not defective, the odds of tossing 10 straight heads are only one in 1,000.

We therefore conclude that the quarters must be different (e.g., the second one has two heads, or is "gimmicked" so that heads comes up more often), and reject the null hypothesis. The *p value* is the probability that the two differences occurred merely by chance (0.001 in this example); for biomedical studies, we usually set the cutoff at 0.05 (5%). This value is called *alpha* (α) and is the probability of a *type I error* (i.e., we proclaim there was a difference when one truly did not exist). As long as *p* is less than α, we reject H_0 and state that the finding is "statistically significant." So, here, we would say that, at the 0.05 alpha level, the two quarters are significantly different.

Remember that this does not prove statistical significance beyond any possible doubt! It still is *possible* to throw 10 straight "heads" with a "normal" quarter—although it is unlikely (the probability of winning the lottery is much less than 0.001, but some extremely lucky person does win all the time). We are merely hypothesizing that it is so improbable that there must be some difference between them. For greater rigor, we can set α to a lower level (e.g., 0.01, 0.001, etc.); but doing this would always require an increased sample size, and would be impractical for most biomedical studies.

If we did find out later that the two quarters were identical (and we wrongly rejected H_0), then we committed a type I error (see the table). Analogous statements in medicine would be: we said there was a difference in the drugs when there was not; we said the patient had cancer when she did not. We also refer to this as a "false positive." We can summarize this in a 2×2 table:

Outcome	Disease Positive	Disease Negative
Test positive	TP, True positive (power, $1 - \beta$)	FP, False positive (type I error, α)
Test negative	FN, False negative (type II error, β)	TN, True negative

Let us now say that we again flipped both quarters 10 times and achieved a comparable result (e.g., 6 heads vs 5 heads—within statistical variance). We would probably conclude that there was no difference and would fail to reject H_0. But if we later found a difference between the quarters, then we have committed a *type II error* (failing to detect a difference when there *was* one). This is the same as saying a patient did not have the disease when he did, the drug was ineffective (when it really was), and so on. Whether or not a type I error is worse than a type II depends on what you are trying to measure (e.g., failing to detect HIV in the blood supply (FN, type II error) is obviously more dangerous than throwing blood away that was erroneously thought to contain HIV (FP, type I error)). However, if you aim for 100% certainty all the time, you could never administer blood products as there is always a chance of a type II error (although it may be remote).

The probability of a type II error (false negative) is referred to as beta (β); another important concept is the quantity $1 - \beta$, which we refer to as *statistical power* (true positive). In other words, are we detecting what we want to detect with our test (the definition of "true positive")? One problem with small studies is that they may lack statistical power; usually we want at least 80% power (0.8). Lack of adequate power is a fundamental issue in that the desired variable cannot be measured accurately. The easiest way to increase statistical power is to increase the sample size.

Also remember that statistical significance may not equal clinical significance. Suppose someone did a study that showed that male doctors who wore patterned ties had better patient outcomes than those who wore solid ties. Logically, this does not make sense, and the difference is likely due to other factors (called "confounders.")

A confounding variable is an extraneous variable that correlates (directly or inversely) with the measured variables. One example of a confounding variable is an old study that linked coffee consumption to pancreatic cancer. Those with this malignancy were found to have consumed more coffee. Therefore, coffee causes pancreatic cancer, right? Let us hold on for a minute. When the data were more closely examined, it was found that those persons with highest coffee consumption also had high rates of cigarette smoking; tobacco use is a proven risk factor for many cancers, including pancreatic adenocarcinoma. Therefore, smoking was the culprit (and the confounder in this case), not coffee itself. Be careful when interpreting data suggesting causality.

PRACTICAL EXAMPLES: NUMBER NEEDED TO TREAT (NNT)

In some of our previous issues we have discussed some basic principles of biostatistics. In this issue we will discuss the effectiveness of a healthcare intervention and the benefits we expect. Usually, this is a treatment with medication, the intent of which is to prevent an undesirable outcome (stroke, diabetic complication, vertebral fracture, etc.).

One such measure commonly used in epidemiological studies is the number needed to treat (NNT), which is the average number of patients who need to be treated in order to prevent one additional bad outcome. Intuitively, we would like the NNT to be as low as possible. For example, suppose we have a new medication to treat hyperlipidemia. We might calculate our NNT to be 30, meaning that we prevent one event (e.g., myocardial infarction) for every 30 patients we treat. This is more ideal than an NNT of 3,000, where we would have to treat a hundred times as many patients for the same benefit.

NNT is important in health economics as well as clinical medicine. NNT is important to pharmaceutical and insurance companies, as it is desirable that the high cost of medication is outweighed by the number of people who would benefit; if NNT is extraordinarily high, it may not be economically feasible to manufacture or pay for the drug.

If the event outcome is serious (death, serious disability, etc.), then a high NNT may be acceptable. Ideally, the NNT would be 1 (every patient given the medication would have elimination of the undesirable event). An example of drugs with very low NNTs includes those for bipolar disorder (most NNTs between 5 and 10). However, a high NNT does not always mean a drug should not be used, especially when the undesirable outcome is severe (e.g., death). Also, such medications often carry side effects (e.g., weight gain), and this must also be considered.

It is possible for the NNT to be a negative number; in this case, we realize the intervention is harmful and we call it the number needed to harm (NNH). To compute the NNT, we must first understand the concept of relative risk. There are two types of risk reduction we will concern ourselves with: relative risk reduction (RRR) and absolute risk reduction (ARR). ARR, put simply, is the difference

between two interventions (how much better or worse the treatment is in reducing the undesired outcome). RRR is a relative or proportional difference. RRR represents the probability of the event occurring relative to that in the placebo group. In contrast, ARR is the difference between event rates over a fixed period of time.

Let us do an example. Suppose a (hypothetical) new drug, utandronate, is being marketed by XYZ Pharma for the treatment of osteoporosis. Phase III clinical trials yield the information we need to calculate our NNT:

Control Group (Placebo) Event Rate (CER)	Utandronate Group (Experimental Event Rate, EER)	RRR (CER − EER)/CER	ARR (CER − EER)	NNT (1/ARR)
0.001	0.0001	(0.001 − 0.0001)/0.001 = 0.9 = 90%	0.001 − 0.0001 = 0.0009	1/0.0009 = 1,111

The NNT is therefore the reciprocal of the absolute risk reduction (1/ARR). This, in many ways, gives more useful results than the RRR. While a 90% reduction in risk seems impressive, it must be put in context of real-world examples; the NNT might still be too large for the intervention to be practical.

Another, nonmedical example of "risk reduction": suppose we see that a jewelry store is selling a wristwatch at a 90% discount (analogous to the "RRR"). This may seem like a good deal until we realize that the original price was $20,000 and the sale price is $2,000. While this may be a fine bargain for some, many people are still not willing to pay $2,000 for a watch, so the benefits are not worth the "risk" (i.e., loss of funds) for many.

Let us imagine another clinical example: suppose a patient with diabetes suffers a small foreign body to his left cornea after metalworking without protective eyewear. His wife searches the Internet and finds that the average infection rate for foreign bodies to the eye is 5% and that topical antibiotics cut this risk by 2/3 in patients with diabetes. He is trying to decide whether or not to go see his physician, as there is cost (time off work and cost of the visit) involved.

He decides to go to the office; after his arrival, we can compute the potential benefit based on the statistics. The risk of infection with no antibiotics (control event rate (CER)) is 0.05 (5%). With antibiotics, the risk is (0.05/3) = 0.017 (1.7%) (remember that the treatment reduces the risk by 2/3, so the risk is

only 1/3 the original). The ARR is 0.05 − 0.017 = 0.033. NNT = 1/ARR = 1/0.033 = 30 patients.

We would therefore need to treat 30 patients with topical antibiotics to prevent one infection. Given the low cost and negligible side effects of topical antibiotics and potential severe outcomes of an untreated eye infection, the choice to treat seems reasonable. It may be "less reasonable" with a very costly drug or one with many side effects. The patient may be willing to accept many adverse side effects for treatment of certain diseases, however (e.g., HIV, where the outcome of no treatment is likely death). This is a relatively easy concept for the patient to understand.

It is also mathematically possible to convert odds ratios to NNT. Remember that an odds ratio is a measure of association between an exposure and an outcome; the OR is the odds that an outcome will occur, given a particular exposure (compared to absence of that exposure). An odds ratio of 1.0 shows no association; OR > 1 is a positive association; OR < 1 a negative one.

To do this, we need to know the patient expected event rate (PEER), which is usually the same as the CER. Calculators for this can be found on the Internet; the equations will not be reproduced here.

Notice that, as the treatment effect becomes more pronounced (i.e., the odds ratio increases), the NNT decreases, which is what we would expect. If the odds ratio is less than 1, there is a negative correlation (treatment produces a worse outcome, not better), and the

Odds ratio	0.5		0.7	0.9	0.95	1.05	1.1	1.3	1.5
Patient expected event rate (PEER)	Number needed to harm (NNH)		NNH	NNH	NNH	Number needed to treat (NNT)	NNT	NNT	NNT
0.001	2,000		3,336	10,010	20,020	20,020	10,010	3,336	2,000
0.0001	20,000		33,336	100,010	200,020	200,020	100,010	33,336	20,000

NNT becomes the NNH. Also notice that, as the event rate decreases, the NNT increases by a reproducible amount.

When reading journal articles, understanding (and calculating, if necessary) the NNT is essential to determine if the intervention is important in your practice. It is also an important tool to help your patients understand. When dealing with patients, it is best to be quantitative and use the NNT rather than RRR (which is dimensionless and more difficult for the average person to put into context with a clinical problem).

REVIEW QUESTIONS

1. For a certain study comparing two different diabetes medications, you find that there is a significant difference between the efficacy of the two; $p = 0.02$ (cutoff $\alpha = 0.05$). However, nine other studies (done by reputable researchers at major universities) have been done on the same two medications and have failed to detect any difference. The patient sample populations studied in your trial are similar to that of the others. The most likely reason that you found a statistically significant difference while others have not is:

   a. You have committed a type I error
   b. You have committed a type II error
   c. Your study has insufficient power
   d. The other studies have significant flaws in design which resulted in no statistical differences
   e. Your study has only a 2% (0.02) chance of providing the correct result

   (a) More than likely, there is no difference in efficacy between the two medications, as nine other well-conducted studies have failed to detect a difference. Your results claim a difference, which is most likely due to a type I error (failing to reject the null hypothesis when it should be rejected). This is the same as a "false positive" laboratory test.

   A type II error (b) is the opposite—stating there was no difference when in fact there was one (a "false negative").

   Insufficient power (c) usually leads to lack of statistical significance, not type I errors.

While it is possible that some of the other trials had flaws (d), it is unlikely that they all were flawed to the extent to give the same result (no difference). The p value of 0.02 means that there is a 2% chance that the difference seen between the two medications was purely due to chance, not that there is a 2% chance of providing the correct result (e). We reject the null hypothesis since our p value is less than our alpha (α) of 0.05 (typical for biomedical studies).

2. A new medication for osteoporosis reduces the risk of hip fracture to 1.5%. The control group fracture rate is 3.5% in the population treated. The NNT to prevent one hip fracture is:

   a. 10
   b. 25
   c. 40
   d. 50
   e. 500

   (d) The risk reduction (RR) is 0.015 and the control event rate is 0.035. The absolute risk reduction is $0.035 - 0.015 = 0.02$ or 2%. The $NNT = 1/ARR = 1/0.02 = 50$.

3. A new study links increased cell phone usage to motor vehicle accidents. Which of the following is a possible confounder that should be considered in interpreting the study?

   a. Cell phone usage distracts the driver and therefore results in more accidents

b. High cell phone users are often teenagers, and therefore likely to be high-risk drivers anyway

c. Cell phone users are also more likely to have consumed alcohol prior to driving

(b) Teens are high-risk drivers anyway, and it might be possible that the increased accident risk is from over-representation by that demographic group, rather than cell phone usage. To be valid, the study should consist of similar (control and event) groups. Answer (a) is the alternative hypothesis and therefore not a confounder. There is no evidence that cell phone usage is linked to alcohol consumption (c).

4. A retrospective study looking at the relationship of lung cancer to smoking is conducted. Part of this study involves patients indicating on a survey how many cigarettes they smoked per day 30 years ago. A potential problem here is that patients may not accurately remember how much they smoked back then. This error is termed:

   a. Confounding variable
   b. Recall or responder bias
   c. Type I error
   d. Interviewer bias

(b) The study's accuracy is dependent on the patient properly recalling events that occurred 30 years ago. Errors in recall usually increase as the interval increases; this is termed recall or responder bias. It is not a confounder (a) as the question is directly linked to the outcome. Interviewer bias (d) results from interviewers probing hard for certain answers, which may alter the subject's response.

5. A scientist reports in his study that 24% of group 1 and 42% of group 2 reported significant adverse effects from treatment with a medication; $p = 0.37$. The best interpretation is:

   a. The true percentage difference is 37%
   b. This result is statistically significant
   c. This result is not statistically significant
   d. This difference in percentages is quite unlikely to have arisen by chance

(c) The p value (0.37) is much higher than the traditional α for biomedical studies (0.05), therefore it is not statistically significant, and likely to have arisen by chance.

Glossary

Acromegaly: Disorder resulting from excess growth hormone in adults.

ACTH (adrenocorticotropic hormone): Protein hormone secreted by the anterior pituitary; results in increased glucocorticoid synthesis.

Addison's disease: Primary adrenal insufficiency, usually caused by autoimmune disease.

Aldosterone: Mineralocorticoid made in zona glomerulosa of adrenal cortex.

Amylin agonists: Analogues of the pancreatic hormone amylin useful as an adjunct to insulin.

Amenorrhea: Condition of absent menses; may be primary (menses never occurred) or secondary (previous menses have stopped).

Anabolic: Metabolic processes that create molecules; occur in well-fed state.

Angiotensin II: Potent vasoconstrictor produced in the liver upon stimulation from renin; trophic hormone for aldosterone secretion.

Antidiuretic hormone (ADH, vasopressin): Posterior pituitary hormone important in water metabolism.

Apolipoproteins: Subcomponents of lipoprotein molecules; various types exist.

Autoimmune disease: Disorders caused by antibodies produced by the body against its own organs.

Becquerel: Unit of radionuclide activity; 1 Ci (curie) = 37 GBq (gigabecquerels).

Beta (β) particle: Electron emitted from an atom's nucleus after decay; negatively charged.

Bile acid sequestrants (resins): Drugs which bind cholesterol in the intestine and prevent its recirculation; useful in hypercholesterolemia.

Calcitonin: Protein hormone made by the parafollicular cells of the thyroid; regulator of calcium metabolism.

Catabolic: Metabolic processes that break down molecules for fuel; useful when organism needs food.

Catecholamines: Hormones derived from tyrosine and secreted by adrenal medulla and other neural tissues, for example, norepinephrine, epinephrine.

Cholesterol: A molecule that plays an important role in atherosclerosis and also serves as a precursor of steroid and sterol hormones.

Chylomicrons: Large, buoyant lipoproteins important in carrying dietary triglyceride to cells.

Colloid: Proteinaceous substance in the thyroid follicle containing thyroglobulin and iodothyronine molecules.

Computed tomography (CT): Uses conventional X-ray beams to produce high-resolution 'cross-sections' of a body part.

Congenital adrenal hyperplasia: Disorder of adrenal enzyme synthesis resulting in accumulation of steroid precursors, with varying deleterious effects.

Cortisol (hydocortisone): Glucocorticoid made in zona fasciculata of adrenal cortex.

Cortisone: Derivative of cortisol.

CRH (corticotropin-releasing hormone): Hypothalamic hormone that stimulates ACTH secretion.

Curie: Unit of radionuclide activity; $1\,Ci = 3.7 \times 10^{10}$ disintegrations per second.

Cushing's disease: Type of Cushing's syndrome caused by an ACTH-secreting pituitary tumor.

Cushing's syndrome: Disorder resulting from excess glucocorticoids.

Cytokines: Mediators secreted by immune cells; important in regulation of many endocrine processes.

Diabetes insipidus: Disorder of excessive thirst and urination resulting from inadequate antidiuretic hormone.

Diabetes mellitus: Disorder of ineffective glucose metabolism.

Dipeptidyl peptidase-4 (DPP-IV) inhibitors: Drugs (e.g., sitagliptin, saxagliptin) which decrease the degradation of incretins such as GLP-1, used as a therapy in type 2 diabetes.

Disorder of sexual differentiation (DSD): Disorder in which gender phenotype may not match genotype (e.g., ambiguous genitalia).

Dopamine: Catecholamine hormone produced by adrenal medulla and other neuroendocrine tissue; inhibits prolactin and TSH secretion.

Endocrine disruptors: Chemicals (often pollutants in the environment) that can interfere with endocrine function in mammals.

Endogenous: Originates from inside the body, for example, endogenous hyperthyroidism.

Epinephrine: Catecholamine hormone produced by adrenal medulla and other neuroendocrine tissue.

Estradiol: Primary estrogen (female hormone); secreted by ovary.

Euthyroid sick syndrome: Condition in which alterations in protein binding lead to low total T3 and/or T4 levels with normal free levels in euthyroid patients.

Exogenous: Originates from outside the body, for example, exogenous corticosteroid ingestion.

Feedback inhibition: Regulatory mechanism; increase or decrease in hormone levels result in appropriate degree of stimulation by trophic hormone.

Fibric acid derivatives: Drugs useful in treatment of hypertriglyceridemia.

Fludrocortisone: Synthetic mineralocorticoid used in treatment of adrenal insufficiency.

FSH (follicle-stimulating hormone): A glycoprotein hormone made by the anterior pituitary gland, important in gonadal regulation.

Gamma rays: High-energy photons emitted from an atom's nucleus after a nuclear event (e.g., ejection of an electron).

Gestational diabetes mellitus: Diabetes which develops during pregnancy.

GHRH (growth hormone-releasing hormone): Hypothalamic hormone that stimulates GH secretion.

Gigantism: Disorder resulting from excess growth hormone in children.

Glucagon: Protein hormone made by pancreatic alpha cells; antagonist to insulin.

Glycogen: Short-term fuel comprised of multiple glucose molecules; stored in liver and muscle.

Glycoprotein: A protein molecule attached to sugars.

GnRH (gonadotropin hormone-releasing hormone): Hypothalamic hormone that stimulates LH and FSH secretion.

Goiter: Enlargement of the thyroid; may be nodular or diffuse.

Graves' disease: Common cause of hyperthyroidism caused by antibodies which mimic TSH action on the thyroid.

Growth hormone (GH): Anterior pituitary hormone important in normal growth and development.

Gynecomastia: Abnormal breast tissue development in males; usually a benign condition.

Hashimoto's thyroiditis: Also called Hashimoto's disease; common endocrine disorder often resulting in goiter and hypothyroidism.

HDL (high-density lipoprotein): Scavenger lipoprotein important in removing cholesterol from cells.

Hermaphrodite: Person containing reproductive organs of both sexes.

Hirsutism: Abnormal terminal (dark) hair growth in women.

HMG-CoA reductase: Rate-limiting enzyme in cholesterol biosynthesis; site of attack of many lipid-lowering drugs.

HMG-CoA reductase inhibitors (statins): Potent inhibitors of cholesterol biosynthesis; useful in lowering LDL cholesterol.

Hydrocortisone: Same as cortisol.

Hyperthyroidism: Any condition resulting in increased thyroid hormone levels.

Hypoglycemia: Condition of decreased serum glucose, resulting in symptoms of hypoglycemia; symptoms resolve after treatment.

Hypogonadism: Condition resulting from decreased sex steroids.

Hypoparathyroidism: Condition of parathyroid hormone deficiency, resulting in hypocalcemia and hypophosphatemia.

Hypothyroidism: Condition where too little thyroid hormone exists.

Incretin mimetic (GLP-1 agonists): Agonist of the GLP-1 receptor useful in the treatment of type 2 diabetes.

Insulin: Protein hormone made by pancreatic beta cells; important in normal glucose metabolism.

Iodothyronines: Thyroid hormones, for example, T4 (thyroxine) and T3 (triiodothyronine).

Kallmann's syndrome: Syndrome of hypogonadotropic hypogonadism resulting from defect in GnRH secretion.

Klinefelter's syndrome: Common cause of hypergonadotropic hypogonadism in males, resulting from 47, XXY chromosomal defect.

LDL (low-density lipoprotein): Atherogenic lipoprotein that carries cholesterol to cells.

Leydig cells: Testicular cells which are the site of testosterone production.

LH (luteinizing hormone): A glycoprotein hormone made by the anterior pituitary gland, important in gonadal regulation.

Lipids: Molecules that provide long-term energy for the body (triglycerides) and other functions; some are atherogenic.

Lipoprotein: Molecule that carries lipids throughout the body.

Magnetic resonance imaging (MRI): Uses high-powered magnetic fields to produce images based on oscillation of hydrogen nuclei.

Meglitinides: Short-acting insulin secretagogues useful in the therapy of type 2 diabetes.

Metformin: Oral diabetes drug that decreases hepatic glucose output and improves insulin sensitivity in patients with type 2 diabetes.

Multinodular goiter: Thyroid gland with two or more nodules; may be euthyroid or toxic.

Nicotinic acid (niacin): Vitamin B3; useful drug for hyperlipidemia in high doses.

Norepinephrine: Catecholamine hormone produced by adrenal medulla and other neuroendocrine tissues.

Nuclear medicine: Science in which radioactive substances given to patients may be used for imaging or therapy.

Osteomalacia: Condition caused by decreased calcium formation in bone.

Osteoporosis: Disorder of decreased bone mass.

Panhypopituitarism: Deficiency of all pituitary hormones.

Paraneoplastic (ectopic) syndrome: Endocrine disorder resulting from secretion of a hormone by a cell type not normally associated with it.

Parathyroid hormone: Protein hormone manufactured by parathyroid glands; important regulator of calcium metabolism.

Parathyroid hormone-related protein: PTH-like protein important in fetal development; may cause hypercalcemia if secreted in certain malignancies.

Polycystic ovary syndrome: Disorder of chronic anovulation resulting in amenorrhea, infertility, and hyperandrogenism.

Positron: β particle with a positive charge.

Precocious puberty: Condition in which puberty commences too early; may be complete (central or true) or incomplete (peripheral).

PRH (prolactin-releasing hormone): Hypothalamic hormone that increases pituitary prolactin production; recently isolated.

Primary endocrine disorder: Defect lies in the target gland itself.

Progesterone: Steroid hormone important in female reproductive cycle.

Prolactin: Anterior pituitary hormone important in mammalian lactation.

Prostaglandins: Hormones formed from fatty acids; play a variety of biological roles.

Protein: A molecule, often large, comprised of many amino acids.

Psuedohermaphrodite: Person whose phenotype (appearance) is opposite that of the genetic sex.

Psuedohypoparathyroidism: Disorder of parathyroid hormone resistance; often occurs with characteristic physical anomalies.

Radioactive iodine: Typically ^{123}I or ^{131}I; usually used as sodium iodide (NaI) in thyroid imaging or treatment.

Rickets: Consequence of vitamin D deficiency in children.

Second messenger: Produced by hormones that bind to cell surface receptors; have biologic effect on nucleus.

Secondary endocrine disorder: Defect lies in the secretion of the trophic hormone for the target gland.

Secretagogue: Substance used in perturbation tests of endocrine function that stimulates hormone secretion.

Sertoli cells: Testicular cells which are the site of sperm production.

SIADH (syndrome of inappropriate antidiuretic hormone secretion): Condition of ADH excess resulting in retention of free water and hyponatremia.

Somatostatin: Hormone produced by hypothalamus and pancreas; inhibitory effects on several hormones.

Spironolactone: Androgen and aldosterone antagonist useful in treating hyperaldosteronism and hirsutism.

StAR (steroidogenic acute regulatory protein): Important in transferring cholesterol to mitochondria for corticosteroid synthesis.

Sulfonylureas: Oral hypoglycemic agent that increased endogenous insulin secretion.

Syndrome X: Syndrome of hyperinsulinemia, hypertension, glucose intolerance, hyperlipidemia, and atherosclerosis.

T3 resin uptake: Indirect measurement of thyroid binding proteins; correlates inversely with protein levels.

Technetium: Man-made radioactive element important in nuclear medicine.

Tertiary endocrine disorder: Defect lies one step higher than the trophic hormone (e.g., hypothalamic dysfunction).

Testicular feminization: Syndrome of androgen resistance resulting in normal female phenotype in a genetic male.

Testosterone: Primary androgen (male hormone); secreted by testis and adrenal gland.

Thiazolidinediones: Insulin-sensitizing drugs useful in the treatment of type 2 diabetes.

Thyroglobulin: Protein upon which thyroid hormones are synthesized and stored in the thyroid follicle.

Thyroid-binding globulin (TBG): Major thyroid hormone transport protein.

Thyrotoxicosis: Condition in which excess thyroid hormone is present in the blood; of endogenous origin.

Thyroxine (T4): Principal hormone secreted by the thyroid gland.

TRH (thyrotropin-releasing hormone): Hypothalamic hormone that increases pituitary TSH production.

Triglycerides: Energy-rich component of adipose tissue.

Triiodothyronine (T3): Most active thyroid hormone; mainly formed by peripheral conversion of T4 in the blood.

Trophic hormone: Hormone that stimulates another hormone's production.

TSH (thyroid-stimulating hormone): A glycoprotein hormone made by the anterior pituitary gland, important in thyroid regulation.

Turner's syndrome: Common cause of hypergonadotropic hypogonadism in females; typical 45XO karyotype, short stature, webbed neck, and infertility.

Tyrosine: Amino acid used as building block of catecholamine and iodothyronine hormones.

Tyrosine kinase inhibitors: Chemotherapeutic agents useful in the therapy of metastatic thyroid cancer.

Ultrasound: Imaging modality using the attenuation of high-frequency sound waves through matter.

Vitamin D: Sterol hormone important in normal calcium absorption from the intestine.

VLDL (very low-density lipoprotein): Triglyceride-rich lipoprotein important in carrying endogenous triglyceride to cells.

X-rays: High-energy photons emitted from an atom's electron shell after a nuclear event.

Index

Page numbers in *italics* refer to Figures; those in **bold** to Tables; those <u>underlined</u> to Definitions.

absolute risk reduction (ARR) 124
ACEIs (angiotensin converting-enzyme inhibitors) 65, 89
achondroplastic dwarfism 17
acromegaly 5, 17–18, *18*, 23, 25, <u>127</u>, <u>128</u>
ACTH (adrenocorticotrophic hormone) 14, 15, 53, <u>127</u>
  Addison's disease 44, 50
  Cushing's syndrome 42, *42*, 43–44
  feedback loops *41*, 41–42
  hypopituitarism 20, 25
  syndrome 118
Action to Control Cardiovascular Disease in Diabetes (ACCORD) trial 63
acute pancreatitis 110
Addison's disease 6, 7, 11, 44–45, 49–51, 53–54, <u>127</u>
  hypercalcemia 82
  polyendocrine disorders 116
  secondary *46*
adenomas, paraneoplastic syndrome 42
ADH (antidiuretic hormone) 2, *2*, 7, 15, 21–26, <u>127</u>
adrenal cortex *40*, 40, *41*, 53
adrenal crisis//shock 45
adrenal endocrinology 1, *40*, 40–42, *41*, 49–51, 53–54
  congenital adrenal hyperplasia 45–47, 53
  incidentaloma *48*, 48–49
  see also ACTH; Addison's disease; Cushing's syndrome
adrenal medulla 47–48
adrenarche (pubarche) 95, <u>105</u>
adrenocortical carcinoma 47
adrenocorticotrophic hormone. *see* ACTH
advanced glycation endproducts (AGEs) 63
adult-onset diabetes. *see* type 2 diabetes
AF (atypical femoral fractures) 86
alcohol consumption, and osteoporosis 84
aldosterone 2, 11, 40, *41*, 46–47, 54, <u>127</u>
aldosteronism, secondary *47*, 47

alendronate 85–86, **86**
alkalosis, metabolic 82. *see also* diabetic ketoacidosis
alpha-glucosidase inhibitors 71, **72**
amenorrhea 19, 24, 100, 103, 104, 106, <u>127</u>
amino acid hormones 2
amiodarone 29
amplification cascades 3, *3*
amylin (human islet amyloid polypeptide) 55, 71
amylin agonists **72**, <u>127</u>
anabolic phase, energy metabolism 54, <u>127</u>
anaplastic thyroid carcinoma 37, 40
androgen insensitivity syndrome. *see* testicular feminization
androgen to estrogen (A:E) ratios, gynecomastia 99–100
androgens 40, 105. *see also* dihydrotestosterone; steroid hormones; testosterone
androgenetic alopecia 95
android obesity 102
andropause 97
angiotensin II *46*, 46, *47*, 47, 54, <u>127</u>
angiotensin converting-enzyme inhibitors (ACEIs) 65, 89
angiotensin receptor blockers (ARBs) 65
ANP (atrial natriuretic peptide) 1, 2, 47
antacids 82, 88, 89
anterior pituitary gland 1, *14*, 14, *15*
antibiotics 51, 70
antibody-mediated endocrine organ destruction. *see* autoimmune diseases
antidepressants, hyperprolactinemia 19
antidiuretic hormone (ADH) 2, *2*, 7, 15, 21–26, <u>127</u>
antihyperglycemic agents, diabetes mellitus therapy 69
antithyroid peroxidase (TPO) 38
apo-B-rich lipoproteins 107, 109, 110
apolipoproteins 107, 108, <u>127</u>

ARBs (angiotensin receptor blockers) 65
arginine vasopressin 2, *2*, *7*, 15, 21–26, 127
ARR (absolute risk reduction) 124
aspart 67, **67**
astronauts, osteoporosis 84
atherosclerosis 27, 107, 109, 110, 112, 115
atorvastatin 111
atrial natriuretic peptide (ANP) 1, 2, 47
atypical femoral fractures (AF) 86
autism/autism spectrum disorders 15
autoimmune atrophic thyroiditis 29
autoimmune diseases 29, 31, 44, 57–58, 127
    diagnosis 10
    hormone deficiency and excess syndromes 6, 7
    polyendocrine disorders 116
    thyroid endocrinology 33
    see also Graves' disease; Hashimoto's thyroiditis; type 1
        diabetes
autonomic neuropathy 64

bad cholesterol. *see* low-density lipoproteins
baldness, male pattern 95
Banting, Fred 66
bariatric surgery 60–61
Bayes' Theorem 121
becquerels 9, 127
beta-blockers 32, 33, 34, 38, 48
beta-hCG (human chorionic gonadotropin) 2, 30, 93,
        97–98
beta lipoproteins. *see* low-density lipoproteins
beta particles 8, 28, 127
biguanides 70
bile acid sequestrants/resins **72**, 111, **112**, 116, **120**, 127
bile acids 106
binding proteins. *see* carrier proteins
biomarkers of disease. *see* genetic markers of disease
bisphosphonates 83, 85–87, **86**, 92, 118
blindness, diabetes mellitus 64
body mass index (BMI) 60
body proportions, abnormal 96–97, *97*, **98**, 104, 106
bone 15, 80, 81, 84, 85, 87, 91. *see also* osteoporosis
bone age (BA) studies 95–96, 105
boys, growth curves *16*, 16
Brassicaceae (brassica family) vegetables 31–32
breast cancer 82, 86, 99
bromocriptine 19, **72**
bruising, exogenous Cushing's syndrome *43*, 43, 53
buffalo hump 43
burn victims 5

cabbage family (Brassicaceae) 31–32
cabergoline 44
cachexia 42
CAH (congenital adrenal hyperplasia) 45–47, 53, 127
calcidiol 80
calcification, ectopic 8
calcitonin 80, 86, 118, 127
calcitriol 80
calcium metabolism 3, 79–80, 88–89, 91–92
    bone 80, 84, 91
    osteoporosis 84–87, *85*, **86**
    regulation *79*
    serum calcium concentration vs. PTH levels
        83–84, *84*
    transport *79*
    vitamin D deficiency 87
    see also hypercalcemia; hypocalcemia
calcium-sensing receptor (CaSR) 80
canagliflozin **72**
candidiasis, mucocutaneous 116
CAPD (continuous ambulatory peritoneal dialysis) 65
car fueling analogy, feedback inhibition 4
carbohydrate counting, diabetes mellitus 68
carbamazepine 22, 23
carcinoid tumors 117
cardiac hormones, sodium metabolism 47
cardiovascular disease 30, 109, 110, 115, **120**
carrier proteins 3, *3*
    calcium *79*, *79*, 91
    lipids 107
    thyroid-binding globulin 34
    thyroxine 28
catabolic phase, energy metabolism 55, 127
catecholamine hormones 2, 3, 4, 5, 47–48, 54, 127. *see also*
        dopamine; epinephrine; norepinephrine
cell membranes 106
cell surface receptors, hormones 3, *3*
central diabetes insipidus 22, 23, 25–26
central obesity 43, 49, 53, 101
certified diabetes educators (CDEs) 69
CGM (continuous glucose monitoring) 69, *69*
children
    diabetes mellitus **10**, 62, 63
    gonadal axis *94*
    testosterone deficiency **98**
chlorpropamide 22, 23
cholesterol 2, 40, *41*, 106, 107, 112, 115, 127
    chemical structure *2*
    clinical trials **120**

exogenous and endogenous pathways *108*, 108–109
 hyperlipidemia 109, 110, 111
cholesterol absorption inhibitors 111, **112**, 115–116
Cholesterol Lowering Atherosclerosis Study **120**
cholestyramine 111, **120**
Chvostek's sign 83, 88
chylomicronemia syndrome 110
chylomicrons 107, *107*, *108*, 109, 111, 115, 127
cigarette smoking, calcium metabolism 84, 86, 89
cinacalcet 81
classical endocrine glands 1
clinical trials 119–120, **120**, 125–26
 number needed to treat 123–125, **124**, **125**
 positive predictive value **121**, *121*, 121–122
 sensitivity and specificity 120–121
 statistical significance 122–123, 125, 126
 type 1/2 errors 122–123, **123**, 125
clofibrate 22, 23
clomiphene citratet 102
'cold' thyroid nodules *35*, 35
colesevelam **72**, 111, 112. *see also* bile acid sequestrants
colestipol 111, **120**
colloids 127
colony-stimulating factors, cytokines 5
computed tomography (CT) 9, 10, 14, *48*, 127
computer analogy, thyrotoxicosis 30
confounding variables 42, 83, 88, 92, 123, 125–126
congenital adrenal hyperplasia (CAH) 45–47, 53, 127
congenital hypothyroidism 29
Conn's syndrome 46
constitutional short stature 16–17, *17*, 25
continuous ambulatory peritoneal dialysis (CAPD) 65
continuous glucose monitoring (CGM) 69, *69*
corneal arcus, hyperlipidemia 110
coronary artery disease 30, 109, 110, 115, **120**
corticosteroids, synthetic. *see* glucocorticoids
corticotropin (adrenocorticotrophic hormone). *see* ACTH
corticotropin-releasing hormone (CRH) 15, 127
cortisol 5, 11, 53. *see also* Cushing's syndrome;
 glucocorticoids; hydocortisone
cortisone 24, 41–42, *41*, 45, 127, 128
cosyntropin (synthetic ACTH) test 11
creatinine clearance 65, 81
cretinism 29
CRH (corticotropin-releasing hormone) 15, 127
CT (computed tomography) 9, 10, 14, *48*, 127
Curie, Marie 8–9
Cushing's disease 7, 42, 44, 45, 49, 53, 118, 127
Cushing's syndrome 4, 42–44, *43*, 49, 53, 117–118, 127

cytochrome P450 oxygenases 40
cytokines 1, 5, 127

dapagliflozin **72**
de Vinci, Leonardo 96
delayed puberty 95, 95–96, **98**
demeclocycline 23
denosumab 86, **86**
deoxycorticosterone (DOC) 45
desmopressin 7, 22
destructive thyroiditis *33*, 33–34, 38, 39
detemir 67, **67**
DEXA (dual-energy X-ray absorptiometry) *85*, 88, 92
dexamethasone 45
dexamethasone suppression test 11, 43
DHA (docosahexaenoic acid) 112
DHT (dihydrotestosterone) 95, 103
Diabetes Control and Complications Trial (DCCT) 63, 77,
 119, 120
diabetes insipidus (DI) 22, 26, 127
diabetes mellitus (DM) 6, 7, 11, *59*, 69, 74–76, 77–78,
 127
 antidiuretic hormone 22
 clinical trials 119–120
 complications 62, 63–66, *64*, *66*
 diagnostic criteria/diagnosis 10, **57**
 epidemiology 58
 genetic markers **10**
 gestations **56**, 61–62, 77, 128
 glucose metabolism 55–59, **56**, *58*, *59*, 63
 growth hormone 18
 lipid disorders 111, 112–113, 115
 monitoring 62, 62–63, 69, *69*, 77
 and obesity 61–62
 prevention and cure 72–73
 secondary 58, 61–62
 team approaches 69
 therapy 66–74, *68*, *69*, *72*. *see also* insulin; type 1
 diabetes; type 2 diabetes
diabetic ketoacidosis (DKA) 65–66, *66*, 74–75, 78
dialysis 65
diet therapy
 diabetes mellitus 67–68, *68*, 78
 lipid disorders 111, 115
 osteoporosis 86, **86**
 see also nutritional deficiencies
differentiated epithelial thyroid cancers 36–37
dihydrotestosterone (DHT) 95, 103
dipeptidyl peptidase-4 (DPP-IV) inhibitors 71, *72*, 78, 128

disorders of sexual differentiation (DSD) 45, 102–103, *103*, 104, 128

DKA (diabetic ketoacidosis) 65–66, *66*, 74–75, 78

DOC (deoxycorticosterone) 45

docosahexaenoic acid (DHA) 112

dopamine 15, 19, 128

dopamine agonists 19, **72**

DPP-IV inhibitors 71, *72*, **72**, 78

drug therapies. *see* pharmacologic agents

dual-energy X-ray absorptiometry (DEXA) *85*, 88, 92

dwarfism, achondroplastic 17

dwarfism, psychosocial 17

dyslipidemia. *see* hyperlipidemia

dyspareunia (painful intercourse) 100

ectopic syndrome. *see* paraneoplastic syndrome

ectopic calcification 8

eicosanoid prostaglandins 2

eicosapentaenoic acid (EPA) 112

endocrine disrupters 128

endocrine pancreas 1

endocrine system/endocrinology 1, 1, 11, 13–14

   disorders 4, 6–8. *see also specific disorders*

   genetic markers of disease **10**, 10

   imaging 8–10, *9*, 14

   immune system interactions 5

   see also hormones

endogenous lipid pathways *108*, 108–109, 115

endogenous thyrotoxicosis. *see* hyperthyroidism

energy supply and storage, hormone function 1–2

environmental triggers

   autoimmune diseases 6, 10

   diabetes mellitus 57, 59

EPA (eicosapentaenoic acid) 112

epidemiology

   diabetes mellitus 56, 58, 72

   number needed to treat 123–125, **124**, **125**

   osteoporosis 84

   primary hyperparathyroidism 80

epinephrine 128

epithelial thyroid cancers 36–37, *37*, 40

epithelial thyroid carcinoma **10**

eruptive xanthomas *110*, 110

erythromycin 64

Eskimos, Greenland 112

estradiol 11, 92, *93*, 93, 105, 128

estrogen agonists 102

estrogen deficiency 100–101, 106. *see also* menopause; osteoporosis

estrogen, male 99

estrogen therapy 21, 84–86, **86**, 91–92, 99, 101

ethnic groups, osteoporosis 84

etomidate 40

eunuchoidal body proportions 96–97, *97*, **98**, 104, 106

euthyroid sick syndrome 5, 128

evidence-based medicine 119. *see also* clinical trials

evothyroxine 21

exocrine glands 1

exogenous Cushing's syndrome 43

exogenous lipid pathways *108*, 108–109, 115

exophthalmos *32*, 32–33

ezetimibe 111, **112**, 115–116

factitious hormone administration 7, 8

   hyperthyroidism 34, 38, 40

     insulin 73–74, 79

Familial Atherosclerosis Treatment Study (FATS) **120**

familial combined hyperlipidemia (FCHL) 109, 115

familial hypercholesterolemia 115

familial hypertriglyceridemia 110

familial paraganglioma 48

familial pheochromocytoma **10**

fasting hypoglycemia 73

fatty acid hormones 2

FCHL (familial combined hyperlipidemia) 109, 115

feedback inhibition 2, 4, *4*, 128

   adrenal gland/hormones *41*, 41–42, *42*

   calcium metabolism 81

   lipid metabolism 108

   testicular function 92

   thyroid hormones 27

female by default hypothesis 93

femoral fractures, atypical (AF) 86

fibric acid derivatives (fibrates) 111, **112**, 116, 128

fight or flight (stress) hormones 15, 40, 47, 53

fine needle aspiration (FNA) biopsy 9, 35, 38, 40, 50

first-pass phenomenon, deficiency syndromes 7

fish oils 112

fludrocortisone 45, 46, 128

follicular thyroid carcinoma 36–37, *37*

follicle-stimulating hormone. *see* FSH

food pyramid, diet therapy *68*

foot problems, diabetes mellitus 64, *64*

football team analogy 1, 3

   adrenal gland/hormones 40

   glucose metabolism 54

   HPA axis 14, 25

   thyroid gland/hormones 26, 27, 31

fragility fractures, bone health 81
Framingham study **120**
Fredrickson classification, hyperlipidemia *109*, 109
FSH (follicle-stimulating hormone) 2, 19, <u>128</u>
  hypogonadism 97–98
  hypopituitarism 20–21
  HPA axis 15
  ovarian function 92–93, *93*
  puberty 94, *94*
  reproductive endocrinology 105

GAD (glutamic acid decarboxylase) 57
galactorrhea 25
gamma radiation 8, 9, <u>128</u>
gastric pacing 64
gastrinoma, multiple endocrine neoplasia syndromes. 117
gastrointestinal system 1, 2
gastroparesis, diabetic 64
gemfibrozil **120**
gender development. *see* disorders of sexual differentiation
genetic markers of disease **10**, 10, 60
  pheochromocytoma 48
  thyroid cancer 40
  thyroid nodules 36
  type 1 diabetes 57–58
genetics
  hypogonadism 97, 98
  hypopituitarism 20
  osteoporosis 84
  polyendocrine disorders 116
gestational diabetes mellitus **56**, 61–62, 77, <u>128</u>
GHRH (growth hormone-releasing hormone) 15, <u>128</u>
gigantism 5, 17–18, *18*, 23, 25, <u>127</u>, <u>128</u>
girls, growth curves *16*
glargine 67, **67**
glomerular filtration rate (GFR), diabetic nephropathy 65
glucagon 1, 55, <u>128</u>
glucagon-like peptide-1 (GLP-1) agonists 69, 71, *71*, **72**, 78, <u>128</u>
glucocorticoids 40, 53. *see also* cortisol *and see below*
glucocorticoids, synthetic 7–8, 41, 46
  Addison's disease 45
  burn victims 5
  congenital adrenal hyperplasias 46
  Cushing's syndrome 43
  exophthalmos 32–33

  osteoporosis 85
  secondary diabetes 61
  short stature 17
  vitamin D-dependent hypercalcemia 83
  see also hydrocortisone
glucocorticoid-remediable aldosteronism (GRA) 46
glucose, chemical structure *54*
glucose intolerance 18
glucose metabolism 1, *54*, 54–55, 74–76, 77
  glucagon *55*, 55
  hyperglycemia 5, 6, 7, 15, 18, 56
  obesity 59–62, **60**, 77
  vitamin D 80
  see also diabetes mellitus; hypoglycemia; insulin
glucose suppression test 5
glucose tolerance test 11, 18
glucose toxicity 59
glucose transporters (GLUTs) 55
glulisine 67, **67**
glutamic acid decarboxylase (GAD) 57
glyburide 70, *70*
glycogen 1–2, 54–55, *54*, <u>128</u>
glycoprotein hormones 2, 3, 4, 30, 93, 97–98, <u>128</u>. *see also* FSH; LH; TSH
GnRH (gonadotropin hormone releasing hormone) 15, <u>128</u>
  amenorrhea 100
  hypogonadism 96, 97
  ovarian function 92–93
  puberty 94, *94*, 96
  testicular function 92
goiter 4, 6, 24, 29, 31, 34, 37, <u>128</u>
gonadotropins 19, 20–21. *see also* FSH; GnRH; LH
gonads 1, 2, 40, 93–94, *94*. *see also* ovarian function; puberty; testicular function
good cholesterol. *see* high-density lipoproteins
GRA (glucocorticoid-remediable aldosteronism) 46
Graves' disease 7, 31, *31*, 34, 38, 39, <u>128</u>
  exophthalmos *32*, 32–33
  polyendocrine disorders 116
  pretibial myxedema *33*
Greenland Eskimos 112
growth, hypogonadal proportions 96–97, *97*, **98**, 104, 106
growth curves *16*, 16–18, *17*, *18*
growth hormone (GH) 11, 14–18, *17*, *18*, 23, 25, <u>128</u>
  hormone measurement 5
  hypopituitarism 21
  pituitary tumors 20

growth hormone (GH) (*continued*)
  treatment of deficiency syndromes 7
  type 2 diabetes mellitus 59
growth hormone-releasing hormone (GHRH) 15, <u>128</u>
growth velocity curves *16*, 16
gynecomastia 99–100, <u>128</u>

hamburger thyrotoxicosis 34
Hashimoto's thyroiditis 11, 29, 38, 39, <u>128</u>
  diagnosis 10
  hormone deficiency syndromes 6
  hormone regulation 4
  polyendocrine disorders 116
heart, endocrine function 1
Helsinki Heart Study **120**
hemochromatosis 6–7
hermaphrodism <u>128</u>. *see also* disorders of sexual
      differentiation
HHM. *see* humoral hypercalcemia of malignancy
high-density lipoproteins (HDL) *107*, 107, 115, <u>128</u>
  exogenous and endogenous pathways 108, *108*, 108,
      109
  hyperlipidemia 109, 110, 111
high-resolution computed tomography 9
hirsutism 45, *101*, 101–102, 106, <u>128</u>
HIV/AIDS 11
HMG-CoA reductase (HMGCR) 108, 111, 115, <u>128</u>
HMG-CoA reductase inhibitors (statins) **112**, *112*,
      115–116, <u>128</u>
HNKS (hyperosmolar nonketotic syndrome) 66
homeostasis. *see* feedback inhibition
honeymoon period, type 1 diabetes *57*, 57, 59, 76
hormone–receptor complexes 3
hormone(s) <u>1</u>, 1, 13–14
  deficiency and excess 4, 6–8, 11, 13–14, 17–18.
      see also specific conditions
  function 1–2
  measurement 5, 5–6
  mechanism of action *3*, 3–4
  regulation *4*, 4
  structure and composition *2*, 2–3
'hot' thyroid nodules 35, *35*
HPA (hypothalamic-pituitary) axis 2, 14–15, 25
  adrenal gland/hormones *41*, 42
  puberty *94*, 94, 96
  thyroid gland/hormones *28*, 39
  see also hypothalamus endocrinology; pituitary
      endocrinology
human islet amyloid polypeptide 55, 71

human chorionic gonadotropin (beta-hCG) 2, 30, 93,
      97–98
humoral hypercalcemia of malignancy (HHM) 82, 83, 89,
      117
hydrocortisone 24, 41–42, *41*, 45, <u>127</u>, <u>128</u>. *see also* cortisol
hyperaldosteronism 7, 46–47, 48, 54
hypercalcemia 80–88*4*, *84*, 89, 91, 116–118
hypercholesterolemia 116. *see also* hyperlipidemia
hyperfunction (hormone excess) 4, 6, 7–8, 11, 13–14,
      17–18. *see also specific conditions*
hyperfunctioning (hot) thyroid nodules 35, *35*
hyperglycemia 5, 6, 7, 15, 18, 56. *see also* glucose
      metabolism
hypergonadotropic hypogonadism 98–99
hyperinsulinemia (insulin resistance) 6, 7, 59, *59*, 102, 109
hyperkalemia 22, 45, 46, 47
hyperlipidemia 109–110, **112**
  clinical trials **120**
  eruptive xanthomas *110*
  Fredrickson classification *109*
  therapy 111–112, *112*
  see also lipid metabolism
hyperosmolar nonketotic syndrome (HNKS) 66
hyperparathyroidism 6, 61, 80–81, *81*, *84*, 85, 88, 91
hyperpigmentation, skin 44, 49–50
hyperprolactinemia 19, 25, *24*
hypertension 47–48, *47*, 50, 54
hyperthyroidism 6, 7, *30*, 30–34, *31*, *32*, *33*, 39, 82, <u>128</u>
hypertriglyceridemia 110, 111, 112, 115, 116
hypocalcemia 81, 83–84, *84*, 87, 88, 91
hypofunction (hormone deficiency) 4, 6–8, 13.
      see also specific conditions
hypoglycemia 7, 8, 15, <u>128</u>
  Addison's disease 45
  glucose metabolism 55, 73–74, *75*, 78–79
  monitoring 62
  unawareness 64
hypogonadal body proportions 96–97, *97*, **98**, 104, 106
hypogonadism 11, 21, 85, 96–100, *97*, 106, <u>128</u>
hypogonadotropic hypogonadism 97–98
hypokalemia 46, 47, 48, 50, 54, 118
hyponatremia 22, 23
hypoparathyroidism 11, 21, 29, 83, *84*, 88, 116, <u>128</u>
hypophosphatemia 87
hypopituitarism 4, 7, **10**, 11, 20–21, 25
hypothalamus endocrinology 6, 14–15, 25
  ADH 21–23
  amenorrhea 100
  GnRH 92–93

tertiary hormone deficiency 20
see also HPA (hypothalamic-pituitary) axis
hypothyroidism 4, 6, 11, 24, 28–30, 34, 38, 39, 128
  atherosclerosis 27
  epithelial thyroid cancers 37
  hyperprolactinemia 19
  hypopituitarism 21
  lipid disorders 109, 115

IAPP (human islet amyloid polypeptide) 55, 71
ibandronate 86, **86**
IDDM (insulin-dependent diabetes). *see* type 1 diabetes
IDL (intermediate-density lipoproteins) 107, *108*, 108
IGF (insulin-like growth factor) 15, 18, 23, 25
ILA (islet cell antibodies) 57
imaging, endocrinology 8–10, *9*, 14
immobilization, osteoporosis 84
immune–endocrine system interactions 5
immunoendocrine syndromes 116. *see also* autoimmune
      diseases
immunosuppressive regimens 7–8
incidentally found adrenal tumors (incidentaloma) *48*,
      48–49
incretin mimetics 69, 71, *71*, **72**, 78, 128
inflammatory responses 2, 6. *see also* cytokines
inhibitory hormones 4
inhibitory tests 11
insulin 1, 6, 7, 70, 73, 77, 128
  diabetes mellitus therapy 66–69, *68*, *69*, 71, 72, 75, 78
  factitious administration 73–74, 79
  glucose metabolism 55, *55*
  pharmokinetics **67**
  pumps *68*, 68–69, 73, 78
  resistance 6, 7, 59, *59*, 102, 109
  secretagogues **72**
insulin-dependent diabetes. *see* type 1 diabetes
insulin-like growth factor I (IGF-I) 15, 18, 23, 25
insulinoma. 117
interferons 5
interleukins 1, 5, 63
intermediate-density lipoproteins (IDL) 107, *108*, 108
intersexuality. *see* disorders of sexual differentiation
intravenressin receptor antagonists 23
iodine atome 26–27
iodine deficiency 29
iodine, radioactive. *see* radioactive iodine
iodothyronine hormones 3, 39, 128
ionized (unbound) calcium 79, *79*, 91
ionizing radiation 9, 10, 14

IQ, and diabetes mellitus 62, 63
iron deficiency anemia 63
islet cell antibodies (ILA) 57

juvenile diabetes. *see* type 1 diabetes

Kallmann syndrome **10**, 97, 129
Kennedy, President John F. 44
ketoacidosis, diabetic (DKA) 65–66, *66*, 74–75, 78
ketoconazole 40
kidney, endocrine function 1. *see also* nephropathy;
      renovascular hypertension
Klinefelter syndrome 98, 100, 104, 129

lanreotide 18
latent autoimmune diabetes in adults (LADA) 57
LDL. *see* low-density lipoproteins
lecithin-cholesterol acyltransferase (LCAT) 108
leukotrienes 2
levothyroxine 21, 24, 29, 30, 38
Leydig cells 25, 92, *92*, 105, 129
LH (luteinizing hormone) 2, 19, 25, 129
  hypogonadism 97–98
  hypopituitarism 21
  HPA axis 14, 15
  puberty *94*, 94
  reproductive endocrinology 92–93, *93*, 105
licorice 47, 50
lipemia retinalis 110
lipid metabolism/lipids 1–2, 106–107, 112–113, 115–116,
      120
  exogenous and endogenous pathways *108*, 108–109,
      115
  lipoproteins *107*, 107–108
  primary disorders *109*, 109–110
  secondary disorders 109–110, 115
  see also hyperlipidemia
Lipid Research Clinics—Coronary Primary Prevention
      Trial (LRC-CPPT)
lipoprotein lipase 107, *108*, 108
lipoproteins *107*, 107–108, 115, 129
local osteolytic hypercalcemia (LOH) 82, 117, 118
lomitapide 110
lorcaserin 60
lovastatin 111, **120**
low-density lipoproteins (LDL) 107–111, *107*, *108*, 115,
      120, 129
low-dose dexamethasone suppression test 43
lung cancer 82, 89, 117–118

luteinizing hormone. *see* LH
lymphocytes, endocrine function 1
lymphocytic hypophysitis 21

Macleod, J.J.R. 66
macroadenomas 19–20, *20*
macroprolactinemia 19
macrovascular diseases 63–66
magnetic resonance imaging (MRI) 9–10, 14, *20*, <u>129</u>
male pattern baldness 95
malignancy-related hypercalcemia 82
MARS (Monitored Atherosclerosis Regression Study) **120**
maturity-onset diabetes of the young (MODY) **10**
medication. *see* pharmacologic agents
medullary thyroid carcinoma (MTC) 37, 40
meglitinides 70, *70*, 78, <u>129</u>
melanocyte-stimulating hormone (MSH) 44
membranes, cell 106
MEN (multiple endocrine neoplasia) 10, **10**, 48, 116–118
menopause 11, 21, 84–85, 97, 100–101, 106. *see also* osteoporosis
menstrual cycle *93*
metabolic alkalosis 82. *see also* diabetic ketoacidosis
metabolic syndrome *59*, 59, 77, 107
metanephrines 48
metformin 70, *70*, 71, **72**, 78, <u>129</u>
methimazole 31–32, 33, 38
metoclopramid 64
microadenomas 19–20
microvascular diseases 63–66, 119
MIF (müllerian inhibitory factor) 93
mifepristone (RU-486) 44
milk-alkali syndrome 82, 89
mineralocorticoid hormones 4, 45, *46*, 46, 53–54. *see also* aldosterone
mipomersin 110
MODY (maturity-onset diabetes of the young) **10**
Monitored Atherosclerosis Regression Study (MARS) **120**
monoclonal antibodies 86, **86**
moon face 43, 53
MRI (magnetic resonance imaging) 9–10, 14, *20*, <u>129</u>
MSH (melanocyte-stimulating hormone) 44
MTC (medullary thyroid carcinoma) 37, 40
mucocutaneous candidiasis 116
müllerian agenesis, primary amenorrhea 100
müllerian inhibitory factor (MIF) 93
multinodular goiter *31*, 31, 34, 38, 39, <u>129</u>
multiple endocrine neoplasia (MEN) 10, **10**, 48, 116–118
multiple myeloma 82

nateglinide 70, *70*
negative predictive value (NPV), clinical trials *121*, **121**, 121–122
neoplasms, gynecomastia 100
nephrogenic diabetes insipidus 22
nephropathy, diabetic 65, 78
neuroendocrinology 1
neurofibromatosis (NF) 48
neurogenic diabetes insipidus 22, 25–26
neuropathy, diabetic 63–64, 75, 78
nicotinic acid (niacin) 111–112, **112**, 116, **120**, <u>129</u>
NIDDM (noninsulin dependent diabetes). *see* type 2 diabetes
nodules, thyroid 3, 14, 15, 34–36, *35*, 38, 40
nomenclature, endocrine disorders 6–7
nonclassical endocrine organs 1
noninsulin dependent diabetes. *see* type 2 diabetes
noninsulinoma pancreatogenous hypoglycemia syndrome (NIPHS) 73
nonpolar (non-charged) hormones 3
norepinephrine 2, 47, 50, <u>129</u>
normal distributions
    bone density 85
    hormone measurement *5*, 5–6
NPH (N) insulin 66, **67**
NPV. *see* negative predictive value
nuclear imaging 8–9, 14
nuclear medicine <u>129</u>
null hypothesis, clinical trials 122
number needed to treat (NNT), clinical trials 123–125, **124**, **125**
nutritional deficiencies
    bariatric surgery 61
    diabetes mellitus 63
    hypocalcemia 83, 88
    see also diet therapy

obesity
    classification **60**
    glucose metabolism 54–55, 59–62, 77
    osteoporosis 84
    polycystic ovary syndrome 102, 106
    and secondary diabetes 61–62
octreotide 18, 34
omega-3 fatty acids **112**, 112
oral contraceptives 101
oral hypoglycemic agents, diabetes mellitus therapy 69, 78
orchidectomy 11

orlistat 60
osteomalacia 87, 129
osteonecrosis of the jaw 86
osteopenia (low bone mass) 85, 87
osteoporosis 43, 81–83, 84, 88–89, 91–92, 129
   calcium metabolism 84–87
   DEXA scans 85, 88, 92
   therapy 85–87, 86, 91–92
ovarian function 92–93, 93, 102, 105
oxytocin 15, 21–23, 23, 25

Paget's disease, bone 87
pancreas 1, 55, 72, 78
pancreatectomy, secondary diabetes 58
pancreatic islet tumors 116–117
pancreatitis 6, 61
panhypopituitarism 20–21, 25, 129
parafollicular (C) cells, thyroid gland 80
paraganglioma syndromes 10
paraneoplastic syndrome 7, 42, 42, 45, 116–118, 129
parathyroid hormone (PTH) 79–80, 81, 83–84, 84, 87, 129.
     see also PTH-rP
parathyroid tumors 80–81, 116–117
patient expected event rate (PEER), clinical trials 124
PCOS (polycystic ovary syndrome) 61, 100, 102, 102,
     106
peptide hormones 3, 4, 7, 47
PET (positron emission tomography) 10
perturbation studies, hormone measurement 5
PGA (polyglandular syndrome) 116
pharmacologic agents
   mineralocorticoids 45, 46
   PTH 83
   statins 112, 112, 115–116, 128
   steroids 7–8, 51
   thyroxine 39
   see also glucocorticoids; hydrocortisone
phentermine 60
phenylthiocarbamide (PTC) 31–32
pheochromocytoma 10, 47–48, 50–51, 54
phospholipids 106, 107, 108, 109
pigmentation, skin 44, 49–50
pituitary adenomas 117
pituitary apoplexy 21, 24
pituitary endocrinology 1, 14, 14, 15, 25
   ADH 2, 2, 15, 21–24, 25–6, 127
   hormone measurement 5
   hormone resistance 34
   hypogonadism 97

hypopituitarism 4, 7, 10, 11, 20–1, 25
   prolactin 14, 15, 18–19
   see also ACTH; growth hormone; HPA axis; TSH
pituitary tumors 19–20, 20, 23–24, 25
   Cushing's syndrome 42, 43–44, 53
   hyperprolactinemia 19, 25
   multiple endocrine neoplasia syndromes 116–117
   secondary hyperthyroidism 34
polycystic ovary syndrome (PCOS) 61, 100, 102, 102, 106
polyendocrine disorders 116–118
polyglandular syndrome (PGA) 116
polypeptide hormones 3, 4, 7, 47
positive predictive value (PPV), clinical trials 121, 121,
     121–122
positron emission tomography (PET) 10
posterior lobe, pituitary gland 14, 14, 21–23
postmenopausal women. see menopause
postpartum thyroiditis 33, 38
postsurgical hypoparathyroidism 88
potassium metabolism 22, 45, 46, 47, 48, 50, 54, 118
pramlintide 71
precocious puberty (PP) 96, 96, 105
prediabetes 56
prednisone 45, 51
pregnancy 5, 6, 19, 24, 42
   diabetes mellitus 56, 61–62, 77, 128
   hyperthyroidism 32
   hypothyroidism 29–30
pregnenolone 40
pretest probability, clinical trials 122
pretibial myxedema 33
primary hormone deficiency syndromes 6, 11, 44.
     see also specific conditions
progesterone 93, 93, 105
proinsulin 55, 55
prolactin 14, 15, 18–19, 20, 21, 25
proptosis (protrusion of the eyes) 32, 32–33
propylthiouracil (PTU) 31–32
prostacyclins 2
prostaglandins 2, 112
protein hormones 2, 2
proteins, binding. see carrier proteins
pseudohermaphroditism. see disorders of sexual
     differentiation
pseudohypoparathyroidism 83, 84, 88
psychogenic polydipsia 22, 26
psychosocial dwarfism 17
PTC (phenylthiocarbamide) 31–32
PTH (parathyroid hormone) 79–80, 81, 83–84, 84, 87, 129

PTH-rP (parathyroid hormone-related peptide) 82, 89, 91, 82, 89, 91, 117, 118, <u>129</u>
PTU (propylthiouracil) 31–32
pubarche 95, <u>105</u>
puberty *94*, 94–96, <u>95</u>, **98**, 105
pumps, insulin *68*, 68–69, 73, 78

radioactive iodine 8, 9, 14, 30, 38
    anaplastic thyroid carcinoma 37
    destructive thyroiditis 33
    follicular thyroid carcinoma *37*
    hyperthyroidism 31, 32
    remnant ablation 36
    thyroid cancer 40
    thyroid scans 28, 35, *35*, 36, 37, 38
radionuclides 8–9, *35*
raloxifene 86, **86**, 99
relative risk reduction (RRR) 124
renin–angiotensin system 46, *46*
renovascular hypertension 47, *47*, 54
reproductive endocrinology 2, 92, 93, 104, 105–106
    amenorrhea 100, 106
    disorders of sexual differentiation 102–103, *103*
    estrogen deficiency 100–101
    gonadal axis, childhood and adulthood *94*
    gonadal differentiation 93–94, *94*
    gynecomastia 99–100
    hirsutism *101*, 101–102, 106
    hypogonadism 11, 21, 85, 96–100, *97*, 106, <u>128</u>
    ovarian function 92–93, *93*, 105
    polycystic ovary syndrome 61, 100, 102, *102*, 106
    puberty *94*, 94–96, 105
    testicular function *92*, 92, 105
    testosterone deficiency **98**
respiratory system 2
retinopathy, diabetic 64, 78, 119
retrospective studies
risedronate 85–86, **86**
RRR (relative risk reduction) 124

St Thomas Atherosclerosis Regression Study (STARS) **120**
saline infusion test 11
salivary cortisol levels, Cushing's syndrome 43
salmon calcitonin 86, 118
Scandinavian Simvastatin Survival Study **120**
Schmidt's syndrome 116
secondary hormone deficiency and excess 4, 6–8, 11, 13–14, 17–18. *see also specific conditions*
secretagogues

insulin 70, 78
    perturbation studies 5
selective estrogen receptor modulators (SERM) **86**, 86, 99
self-blood glucose monitors *62*, 69, 77
sensitivity, clinical trials <u>120</u>, 120–121, <u>121</u>
Sertoli cells *92*, 93, 105, <u>129</u>
sex-hormone binding globulin (SHBG) 3, 97, 98–99
sex steroids 15, 93–99, *94*, *97*, 105–106. *see also* reproductive endocrinology
sexual differentiation disorders. *see* disorders of sexual differentiation
SGLT2 (sodium-glucose transport protein) **72**
Sheehan's syndrome 21
short stature, growth hormone deficiency 16–17
SIADH. *see* syndrome of inappropriate antidiuretic hormone
signaling molecules, lipids 106–107
silent thyroiditis 33
simvastatin 111, **120**
single-photon emission computed tomography (SPECT) 9
sitagliptin 71
skin pigmentation 44, 49–50
small cell lung carcinoma 22, 117–118
smell, sense of 97
smooth muscle contraction 2
sodium metabolism 2, 22, 23, 45, 46, 47
somatomedin C (insulin-like growth factor) 15, 18, 23, 25
somatostatin 15, 18
specificity, clinical trials <u>120</u>, 120–121, <u>121</u>
SPECT (single-photon emission computed tomography) 9
squamous cell lung carcinoma 82, 89
STARS (St Thomas Atherosclerosis Regression Study) **120**
statins. *see* HMG-CoA reductase inhibitors
statistical significance, clinical studies 122–123, 125, 126
steroid hormones 2, 3, 40, 106. *see also* sex steroids
steroid medication 7–8, 51
steroidogenic acute regulatory protein (StAR) 40
stimulatory hormones 4, 6, <u>130</u>
stress hormones 15, 40, 47, 53
striae (stretch marks), Cushing's syndrome *43*, 43, 53
subacute thyroiditis 33
sulfonylureas *70*, *70*, 71, 78
suppressive tests 11
syndrome of inappropriate antidiuretic hormone (SIADH) 22–23, 26, 117, 118
syndrome X *58*, <u>130</u>
synthetic agents. *see* pharmacologic agents

T3. *see* triiodothyronine

T4. *see* thyroxine

tall stature 17–18, *18*, 23. *see also* acromegaly

Tanner stages, puberty 95

TBG (thyroid-binding globulin) 3, 34, 130

team approaches, diabetes mellitus therapy 69

technetium 8, 14, 130

tendon xanthomas 110

teriparatide 86, **86**

tertiary endocrine disorders 6, 20, 130. *see also specific conditions*

testicular function, reproductive endocrinology 92, *92*, 105

testosterone 25, 40, 130
  deficiency syndromes 7, *98*, 98–99
  gonadal differentiation 93–94
  hypogonadism 96, 97
  hypopituitarism 21
  ovarian function 92
  puberty 94, 95

thiazolidinediones (TZDs) 70–71, **72**, 78, 102, 130

thioureas 31–32

thromboxanes 2

thyroglobulin 27, 34, 36, 37, 130

thyroid-binding globulin (TBG) 3, 34, 130

thyroid cancer survey 36

thyroid follicle 26, 27

thyroid endocrinology 1, 26–27, 37–38
  epithelial thyroid cancers 36–37
  factitious hormone administration 8
  hormone synthesis 27
  hypopituitarism 20
  medullary thyroid carcinoma 37
  nodules 34–36, *35*, 38
  regulation 27–28, *28*
  release of preformed thyroid hormone 33
  thyroid follicle structure 26, 27
  thyrotoxicosis 30–34, *31*, *32*, *33*
  see also Hashimoto's thyroiditis; hyperthyroidism; hypothyroidism; thyroxine; triiodothyronine

thyroid peroxidase (TPO) 27

thyroid scan 28, 35, *35*, 36, 37, 38, 39

thyroid storm 34

thyroid-stimulating hormone. *see* TSH

thyroid-stimulating immunoglobulin (TSIg) 31

thyroidectomy 4, 11, 29

thyroiditis, subacute 33

thyrotoxicosis 30, 30–34, 39–40, 130

thyrotropin. *see* TSH

thyrotropin-releasing hormone. *see* TRH

thyroxine (T4) 2, 11, 26–30, *31*, 38, 130
  chemical structure *26*
  destructive thyroiditis *33*, 33–34, 38, 39
  hormone measurement 6
  mechanism of action 3
  secondary hyperthyroidism 34
  synthetic 39

toxic multinodular goiter 31, *31*, 31, 38, 39

TPO (thyroid peroxidase) 27

transcortin, binding protein 3

transforming growth factors 5

TRH (thyrotropin-releasing hormone) 15, 19, 27–28, *28*, 130

tricyclic antidepressants 64

triggers, environmental. *see* environmental triggers

triglycerides 106–112, *106*, *108*, 115, 130

triiodothyronine (T3) 2, 26, 27, 28, 39, 130
  chemical structure *26*, *106*
  destructive thyroiditis *33*
  hyperthyroidism 30, *31*
  hypothyroidism 29
  mechanism of action 3

TRH (thyrotropin-releasing hormone) 15, 19, 27–28, *28*, 130

troglitazone 71

trophic hormones 4, 6, 130

Trousseau's sign 83

TSH (thyroid-stimulating hormone) 6, 7, 25, 38, 39, 130
  epithelial thyroid cancers 37
  hyperprolactinemia 19
  hyperthyroidism 30, 31
  hypopituitarism 20, 21
  hypothalamic–pituitary axis 14, 15
  secondary hyperthyroidism 34
  and thyroid gland/hormones 26, 27–28, *28*, 29, 30

tumor necrosis factor 5, 63

tumors, hormone deficiency and excess syndromes 7

Turner syndrome 98, 99, 100, 104, 106, 130

twin studies
  autoimmune diseases 10
  diabetes mellitus 57–58, 59

two-cell concept of ovarian steroidogenesis *93*, 102, 105

type 1 diabetes (insulin-dependent diabetes) 6, 11, 59, 77, 78
  clinical trials 119
  epidemiology 56
  glucose metabolism 55, **56**, 56–58, *57*
  polyendocrine disorders 116

type 1 diabetes (insulin-dependent diabetes) *(continued)*
    prevention and cure 72, 73
    therapy 7, 66–67
type 1/2 errors, clinical studies 122–123, **123**, 125
type 2 diabetes 4, 7, 11, 58–59, *59*, **72**, 77
    clinical trials 119
    epidemiology 56
    glucose metabolism 55, **56**
    lipid disorders 107, 109, 110
    monitoring 63
tyrosine 2, *2*, 27, 47, 130
tyrosine kinase inhibitors 130
TZDs (thiazolidinediones) 70–71, **72**, 78, 102, 130

ultrasound imaging *9*, 9, 14, 130
    thyroid nodules 28, *35*, 35, 36
United Kingdom Prospective Diabetes Study (UKPDS)
        63, 77, 119
United States, diabetes mellitus 56
urine tests
    diabetes mellitus monitoring 62
    hormone measurement 5, 43, 48

vanillylmandelic acid (VMA) 48
vasopressin. *see* arginine vasopressin
very low-density lipoproteins (VLDL) 107–111, *107*, *108*,
        115, 130
virilization disorders 45, *101*, 101
vitamin B (niacin) 111–112, **112**, 116, **120**, 129
vitamin D 80, 81, 85, 86, 87, 91, 130
vitamin D-dependent hypercalcemia 82
von Hippel–Lindau disease (VHL) 48

Wadlow, Robert 17

xanthelasma 110
X-linked hypophosphatemic rickets **10**
X-rays (roentgenograms) 8, 14, 85, 130

zoledronic acid **86**, 86, 118
Zollinger–Ellison syndrome 117
zona fasciculata *40*, 40, 41, 46
zona glomerulosa *40*, 40, 46
zona reticulata 41

Printed and bound by CPI Group (UK) Ltd, Croydon, CR0 4YY